DID YOU KNOW THAT...

❖ Lung and bronchial congestion can be relieved with a mouthwatering meal of Soba Noodles with Mustard Greens or Bean Curd Cubes with Chicken Sauce?

❖ You can help prevent heart, eye, and kidney disease related to diabetes by eating foods high in omega-3 fatty acids like Steamed Pumpkin with Gingered Honey or Chicken Cubes with Lichee and Plum Sauce?

❖ Tea, taken internally or externally, can help combat the herpes virus because it contains the amino acid lysine?

❖ Eating a dish like Eggplant with Hot Bean Paste can help reduce the swelling of hemorrhoidal tissues?

❖ Cooling, salty foods like Mussels Steamed in Rice Wine can help facilitate proper body fluid movement, and thus alleviate PMS?

MAKE MEALS YOUR MEDICINE!

CHINESE HEALING FOODS

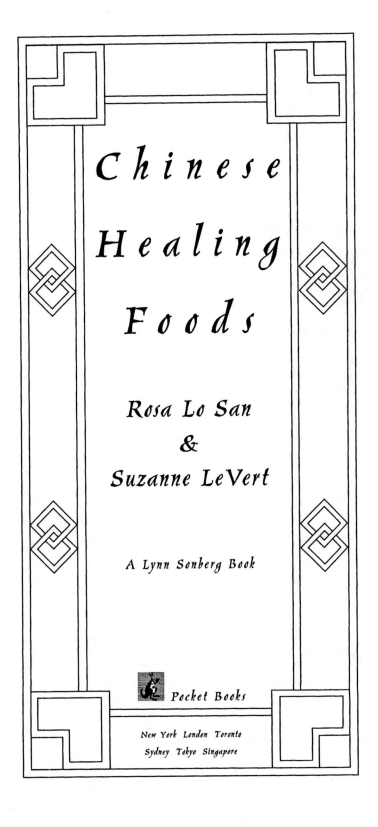

Chinese Healing Foods

Rosa Lo San
&
Suzanne LeVert

A Lynn Sonberg Book

Pocket Books

New York London Toronto
Sydney Tokyo Singapore

An *Original* Publication of POCKET BOOKS

 POCKET BOOKS, a division of Simon & Schuster Inc.
1230 Avenue of the Americas, New York, NY 10020

Copyright © 1998 by Lynn Sonberg

All rights reserved, including the right to reproduce
this book or portions thereof in any form whatsoever.
For information address Pocket Books, 1230 Avenue
of the Americas, New York, NY 10020

Library of Congress Cataloging-in-Publication Data

Ross, Rosa Lo San.
    Chinese healing foods/Rosa Lo San & Suzanne LeVert.
      p.   cm.
    Includes index.
    ISBN: 0-671-52799-1
      1. Diet therapy—Recipes. 2. Cookery, Chinese. 3. Medicine,
    Chinese.   I. Title.
    RM219.R737 1998
    615.8'54'0951—dc21   98–16083
                                                                          CIP

First Pocket Books trade paperback printing September 1998

10   9   8   7   6   5   4   3   2   1

POCKET and colophon are registered trademarks of Simon & Schuster Inc.

Cover design by Jeanne M. Lee
Cover illustration by Lilly Lee
Text design by Meryl Sussman Levavi/digitext, inc.

Printed in the U.S.A.

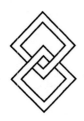

Contents

INTRODUCTION: Food as Health   1

Part I

Healthy Eating: An East/West Perspective   5

CHAPTER ONE: The Yin and Yang of Health   7

CHAPTER TWO: The Healing Properties of Food   29

CHAPTER THREE: Preparing Your Kitchen   47

Part II

An East/West Guide to Common Ailments   61

Anemia   64
Arthritis and Rheumatism   67
Back Pain   71
Bad Breath   73
Bronchitis   75
Candidiasis (Yeast Overgrowth)   77
Chronic Fatigue   80
Cold Sores   82

Colds and Coughs   84

Constipation   86

Diabetes   88

Diarrhea   91

Dizziness   94

Ear Infections   95

Flatulence   97

Flu   99

Hay Fever   102

Headache   104

Hemorrhoids   106

Hepatitis   108

Herpes Simplex Type 2 (Genital Herpes)   110

Hypertension   112

Indigestion   115

Insomnia   118

Menopausal Symptoms   120

Menstrual Problems   122

Nausea   125

Pain, Chronic   127

Psoriasis   130

Sinus Infections   132

Urinary Tract Infections   134

Part III

Chinese Healing Foods: The Recipes   137

Beverages   141

Green Tea   141

Ginger Tea   142

Soups   143

Basil Coconut Soup with Peppermint Sprigs   143

Beef Essence   145

Fishball Soup   146
Ginseng Chicken Soup   147
Vegetarian Hot and Sour Soup   148
Spinach and Bean Curd Soup   149
Sweet Potato Soup   150
Cold Tomato and Ginger Soup   151
White Fungus (Snow Fungus) in Rich Chicken Broth   152
Winter Melon Soup   153

Vegetables   155

Bean Curd Cubes with Chicken Sauce   155
Steamed Stuffed Bitter Melon   156
Bok Choy with Garlic   158
Broccoli with Sesame Dressing   159
Buddha's Delight with Dried Bean Curd Sticks   161
Eggplant with Hot Bean Paste   162
Kohlrabi with Swiss Chard Ribbons   164
Steamed Pumpkin with Gingered Honey   165
Slivered Radish and Cilantro Salad   166
Silk Squash with Oyster Sauce   167
Yam or Taro Root Braised with Nam Yue   168

Fruit   169

Kumquats in Perfumed Syrup   169

Rice and Noodles   171

Cellophane Noodles with Chinese Celery and
    Flowering White Cabbage   171
Basic Congee   173
Ginkgo Nut and Bean Curd Stick Congee   174
Lo Mein with Mushrooms   175
Soba Noodles with Mustard Greens   177
Brown Rice with Mung Bean Sprouts and Cabbage Ribbons   178
Coconut Sweet Rice   179

Meat   181

Hoisin Beef with Red and Green Peppers   181

Soybean Sprouts with Beef   182
Spicy Lamb with Wide Rice Noodles   183
Pork Liver with Garlic Chive Flowers   185
Braised Pork with Black Bean Sauce   186
Five-Spice Pork with Nam Yue   187

Fish and Seafood 188

Steamed Carp on Mustard Greens   188
Clams and Mussels in Black Bean Sauce   189
Fish-Filled Wontons   190
Fish with Lemon Sauce   192
Fish Poached with Rice Wine Sauce   193
Mussels Steamed in Rice Wine   195
Oyster, Mushroom, and Bean Curd Stew   196
Oysters Steamed in Egg Custard   197
Scallops with Long Beans   198
Shrimp Wrapped in Seaweed   199
Squid with Thin Wheat Noodles in Spicy Sauce   200

Poultry 202

Steamed Chicken "Cake"   202
Chicken Cubes with Lichee and Plum Sauce   203
Chicken Legs with Pineapple and Mandarin Peel   205
Chicken with Walnuts   206
Braised Duck with Cinnamon, Garlic, and Bamboo   208
Five-Spice Roast Duck   209

Eggs 211

Steamed Custard with Garlic Chives and Shrimp   211
*Egg White Crab "Omelet" with Button Mushrooms
    and Bean Sprouts*   212

RESOURCE GUIDE   215

GLOSSARY   221

INDEX   231

Chinese

Healing

Foods

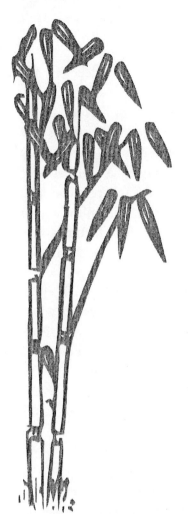

Food as Health

As the twenty-first century approaches, Americans are living longer than ever before—approximately twenty years longer than we did at the beginning of the twentieth century. Today most of us can expect to survive well into our seventies. As a nation, we remain one of the richest on Earth, overflowing with technological and natural resources. Medical science has advanced to the point where we can make a sophisticated x-ray or other imaging technique of an idea being launched in the brain, stop a cancer cell in its tracks, and correct an intricate imbalance of hormones with a simple pill. Indeed, every day we learn a little more about the way the human body works and what we need to do to keep it up and running well. Our supermarkets and refrigerators are overflowing with a wide variety of delicious and nutritious foodstuffs.

Yet something is missing, something is out of balance. At the same time we enjoy these incredible advantages, many of us suffer from undermining physical and emotional ailments that disrupt our lives. Chronic diseases like arthritis, allergies, and diabetes are on the rise, and more than one half of all Americans are overweight. Nearly 10 million American men and women will suffer one or more episodes of major depression during their lifetimes, and another 15 million will experience panic attacks or other symptoms of anxiety.

Without question, the typical American diet may well lie at the heart of many of these problems. "You are what you eat" may be a cliché, but like many clichés, it is one with a great deal of merit. Food provides the body with the raw materials it needs to function properly. Without those ingredients health problems can, and often do, develop. In addition, the anxiety many of us feel over what we eat very often complicates the issue, both because we tend to choose the wrong foods when we're anxious and because our bodies do not digest food or use its energy properly when we're in this state.

In recent decades, many Americans have been looking to Asia for potential solutions to their health problems—as well as for inspiring taste treats. In general, Chinese medicine and its cousins in India and Tibet concentrate more on natural remedies, such as herbs and nutrition, and less on man-made pharmaceuticals than Western medicine. Furthermore, and perhaps more importantly, these remedies are not meant simply to ease a certain symptom or "cure" a specific infection, but rather to reestablish a whole-body balance, to bring the body and the spirit back into proper alignment, an alignment and balance the Chinese call health. And that's the way these cultures tend to look at diet and nutrition—as part and parcel of a whole and balanced way of life and living.

Most Americans, its seems, have been waging a war against food for decades. Food isn't to be enjoyed or savored, but picked apart to see what ingredients it has that might harm us. We completely avoid fat, sugar, red meat, and eggs—until we miss the flavors and textures so much that we completely abandon our good intentions and head directly for the nearest fast-food restaurant or junk-food store aisle. It is this "love–hate, feast or famine" attitude toward food that lies at the heart of many of our chronic health problems.

Fortunately, we're beginning to understand, as Asian cultures have for centuries, that balance and moderation are the keys to both good health and good eating. The Chinese recipes in this book are tasty, healthy, and include a wide variety of vegetables, fruits, meats, and grains, all served in moderate but satisfying portions. Furthermore, you'll see that each food has particular qualities that work to keep your body and soul in harmony and in balance. By matching those qualities to your own physiological needs, you can prevent disease from occurring as well as alleviate health problems when they do arise.

In this book's three parts you will learn just how westerners and easterners approach food and ailments differently and also find recipes that will help you incorporate the healing properties of Eastern foods into your diet quickly and easily. In Part I, you'll learn about the way traditional Chinese medicine looks at health and healing, and how diet and nutrition fit into the picture. You'll also find out what kinds of food and kitchen equipment it's helpful to have on hand when you cook the Chinese way. We'll also explain some Chinese cooking techniques to get you started. In Part II, we discuss some thirty different conditions, including arthritis, indigestion, psoriasis, and urinary tract infections. We'll show you how both Western and Eastern medicine consider each problem, and then we'll discuss some of the most effective nutritional remedies— ones that you can prepare in your own kitchen—for it. Part III provides you with recipes for fifty-six delicious, nutritious Chinese dishes. You'll learn what types of illnesses the recipes may help to alleviate and why, as well as receive easy-to-follow preparation instructions. A Resource Guide that includes a list of mail-order houses for fresh food, spices, and herbs as well as other books about the principles of Chinese health and healing will help you stock your kitchen and library.

Needless to say, this book does not provide sure "cures" for any illness. If you feel ill, see a physician for a diagnosis and, if necessary, medical treatment. We do, however, provide you with a unique opportunity to prepare and enjoy healthy Chinese dishes while learning about China's ancient medical secrets and how they might apply to and improve your life and lifestyle.

Enjoy!

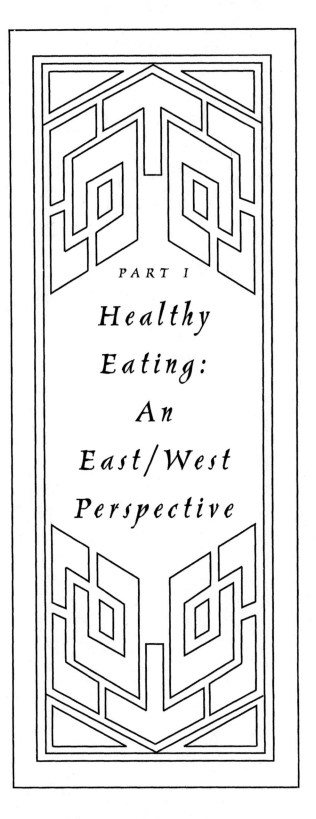

PART I

Healthy Eating: An East/West Perspective

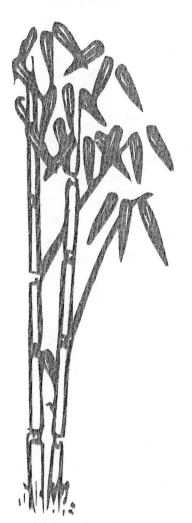

CHAPTER ONE

The Yin and Yang of Health

*I*T WAS LESS THAN THIRTY years ago that most Americans gained their first glimpse of the remarkable tradition of Chinese medicine, which now represents the most popular alternative form of healing in the United States. In 1972, President Richard Nixon made the first official U.S. government trip in nearly three decades to the Chinese capital of Beijing. A few months before that historic visit, appendicitis requiring immediate surgery struck *New York Times* reporter James Reston, who was in China preparing for the president's visit. Instead of administering pharmaceutical anesthetics, his Chinese surgeons used acupuncture to control the pain during and following the procedure. Reston wrote extensively about the successful and pain-free operation he underwent, fascinating readers in this country and throughout the West.

Since that time, interest in acupuncture and other facets of Chinese medicine and philosophy has continued to grow, especially during the 1980s and 1990s, when a new spiritualism converged with people's desire to maintain health and fitness in more natural and balanced ways. Today, with proper nutrition and diet among our greatest medical concerns, China's perspective on nutrition to prevent disease and restore health has special resonance. Because Americans have always enjoyed the rich textures and unique flavors employed in Chinese cooking, finding ways to make this cuisine more healthful and healing offers an additional appeal to the millions of amateur chefs among us.

Chinese medicine appeals to many of us because of its holistic approach. Chinese healers view the human body as an integral part of nature, and see healing as a natural process we can foster by eating and living well. This point of view is one that Western medicine is only just now beginning to accept. In their groundbreaking book called *Between Heaven and Earth,* Harriet Beinfeld and Efrem Korngold, two Western health professionals, described the difference between Western and Eastern philosophies of health and healing very succinctly. Western culture, they wrote, tends to view physicians as "mechanics" and the human body as a "machine." In this view, each separate system, organ, and process within the body works almost completely independently of the others. For instance, we think of the circulatory system as a "plumbing system" with the heart acting as a mechanical pump that pushes blood through the pipes of veins and arteries. We liken the nervous system to a vast communications network made up of electrical connections just like the telephone system. Diseases represent malfunctions of this machine, and to fix the part that's broken is the ultimate goal of medicine. Finding out why it broke down or how this weakness affects the rest of the body is often a secondary consideration at best.

Furthermore, Western medicine historically views the mind—

thoughts, emotions, and perceptions—as being quite separate from the body. The way we feel about life has little or no bearing on our physical health, so this thinking goes, and emotional diseases, like depression, cannot possibly trigger what we consider to be a physical problem, like the flu or heart disease. As you'll see, this is in sharp contrast to the Eastern view of the body, mind, and spirit as one entity, intertwined and interdependent.

The good news is that East and West are beginning to merge their traditions and share the knowledge each has about the human body and how to maintain its health. China, for instance, has borrowed Western surgical techniques and the use of antibiotics and other pharmaceuticals effective against injury and acute infections. At the same time, the United States is beginning to accept the Chinese philosophy of holistic medicine in which the body, mind, and spirit work together as one and therefore has become more focused on the preventive measures such a view fosters.

The Chinese philosophy of holistic medicine has a long and complex history. In the third century B.C., a group of healers in China compiled a text known as *The Yellow Emperor's Classic of Internal Medicine.* This first major treatise on traditional Chinese medicine (TCM) outlines an approach to living a healthy, balanced life still practiced by more than a quarter of the world's population. Throughout the centuries, other healers have added to and adapted its message. It is a complex, all-encompassing philosophy based on spiritual tenets as well as medical theories. As you'll see in Chapter 2, nutrition and the healing properties of food form an integral part of the Chinese approach to health and healing.

Before we explore how food fits into the TCM picture, it's important that you gain at least a cursory appreciation of the fundamentals of this intricate system of beliefs and prescriptions. (The Resource Guide on pages 215 to 220 provides a list of books about all aspects of TCM. Should you decide to investigate TCM further, reading one or more of these texts will help broaden and deepen your knowledge.)

• *A Traditional Chinese Medicine Primer*

At its heart, TCM holds that all of humanity, and each individual human, is part of a larger creation—the universe itself. Each of us is subject to the same laws that govern all of nature: we exist as equals with the stars, planets, animals, trees, oceans, and soil. It is no accident that natural images often come into play as you read about this philosophy. TCM refers to the flows of bodily fluids and energy as channels and rivers, and the state of the body as a whole in terms of natural phenomena: cold, heat, dampness, dryness, and wind.

According to Chinese philosophy, human beings represent the juncture between heaven and earth and thus a fusion of cosmic and earthly forces. Indeed, human beings *are* nature, and as such are subject to the same cyclic patterns, the same ebbs and flows, as the seasons and the tides. The states of the universe, the planet, the nation, and each individual human body are all connected by a unified system known as the *Tao,* or the Way. According to the *Tao,* when any part of this unified whole becomes unbalanced, natural disasters, such as floods or droughts, or human disease may occur. In TCM what injures the earth injures each of us and vice versa, and efforts to heal the human body work to foster the health and well-being of the entire universe.

The Divine Balance of Yin and Yang

In Chinese medicine, health is determined by one's ability to maintain a balanced and harmonious internal environment. Balance—in health and all things—is expressed through the principle of yin/yang. Yin and yang are two dynamic forces that together create everything in the universe.

The Chinese character for yin translates as "the dark side of the mountain," while the one for yang means "the bright side of the mountain." Yin has connotations of cold, dark, and wet, while yang is warm, bright, and dry. Yin is quiet, static, and inactive, while yang is dynamic, active, and expansive.

Every object, condition, and situation can be described as being yin or yang or being *relatively* more or less yin or yang. In other words, it helps to understand yin/yang as a process rather than as a static definition. Going back to the image of the mountain, for instance, the dark side of the mountain is yin in relation to the sunny yang side. As the sun rises and moves across the sky, however, the morning warmth and light it sheds on one slope shifts slowly to the other in the afternoon. Yin becomes yang and yang becomes yin as day becomes night.

Here are some other yin/yang associations:

Yang	Yin
Light	Dark
Heaven	Earth
Sun	Moon
Day	Night
Spring	Autumn
Hot	Cold
Male	Female
Fast	Slow
Up	Down
Outside	Inside
Fire	Water
Wood	Metal

According to Chinese medicine, the human body is divided into yin and yang as follows: The internal region is yin, the external yang. The tendons and bones are yin, while the skin is yang. Yin stands for the storage of energy, while yang stands for activity. Certain organs are considered yin (the heart, liver, lungs, bones, and kidneys) while others are yang (intestines, gallbladder, and skin).

When it comes to disease, yin and yang are used to describe two basic patterns of change. When yin is too strong, yang becomes diseased. When yang proliferates, yin suffers. When yin is deficient, the body and its organs become too hot; when yang is deficient, there will be symptoms of chill and cold.

A primary goal of treatment for any condition, therefore, is to restore the body's balance of yin and yang, to even out heat and cold, dampness and dryness, activity and rest. According to *The Yellow Emperor's Classic of Internal Medicine,* "A hot disease should be treated by cold herbs, a cold disease should be treated by hot herbs...Yin should be treated in a yang disease, yang should be treated in a yin disease." As you'll see in Chapter 2, each food also has more yin or yang qualities, and thus a prescription in Chinese medicine often has a nutritional component.

In order for yin/yang balance to exist—in your body or in the universe—energy, or *qi,* must flow unimpeded and in sufficient quantities throughout the entire system.

Qi: The Life Force

According to TCM, qi is the energy essential for life. All functions of the universe, as well as those of your own body and mind, are manifestations of qi. Your health, therefore, depends on a sufficient, balanced, and uninterrupted flow of qi. Qi circulates through the body along a continuous circuit of pathways known as *meridians.* These meridians flow along the surface of the body and through the internal organs. When you are healthy, you have an abundance of qi flowing smoothly through the meridians and into and out of the organs, allowing your body to function in harmony and balance.

Qi is the source of every aspect of body activity and movement. It is responsible for maintaining normal body temperature and protecting the body from invasion by external factors such as heat, cold, and damp, and is crucial in transforming food and air into other vital substances the body needs. Qi is what allows yin/yang balance to be maintained in the body and in the universe.

When too much qi is evident in an organ or system of the body, the disease that occurs is referred to as an *excess condition*. Conversely, when there is too little qi, a *deficient condition* develops. When qi is deficient, the body tends to decline. Many chronic diseases, like anemia and arthritis, are considered deficient conditions. When qi is in excess, on the other, it tends to become blocked in certain organs or areas, causing swelling, stagnation, and sluggishness. A goal of treatment for any disease, therefore, is to reestablish proper qi energy and flow throughout the body.

Both yin/yang and qi exist in a larger context called the Five Elements, a dynamic representation of nature and the cycle of life.

The Five Elements: A Circle of Nature

The principle of the Five Elements (known as *Wu Hsing* in Chinese) offers a coherent structure to the flow of qi and the balance of yin and yang. It links together the seasons of the year, the aspects of nature, and even your body's organs and bodily processes. By following the Five Elements system, a practitioner of Chinese medicine prescribes treatment to alleviate symptoms and cure disease, linking specific foods, herbs, and acupuncture points to the restoration of yin/yang and qi.

The Five Elements are Wood, Fire, Earth, Metal, and Water. As manifestations of yin and yang, the Five Elements are the fundamental forces of nature whose constant transformations and interactions make all life possible. Just as all matter is made up of yin and yang, so does each thing contain all Five Elements in various proportions.

Indeed, the Five Elements system is best understood as a creative cycle, with each phase nourishing and promoting the activities of the next. All change—in the universe and in your body—occurs in five distinct stages. Each of these stages is associated with a particular time of year, a specific element in nature, and a pair of organs in the body. Here is a quick rundown of these associations:

	Wood	Fire	Earth	Metal	Water
Season	Spring	Summer	Late summer	Autumn	Winter
Direction	East	South	Center	West	North
Climate	Wind	Heat	Dampness	Dryness	Cold
Color	Blue/green	Red	Yellow	White	Blue/black
Taste	Sour	Bitter	Sweet	Pungent	Salty
Yin organ	Liver	Heart	Spleen-pancreas	Lungs	Kidney
Yang organ	Gallbladder	Small intestines	Stomach	Large intestines	Bladder
Emotion	Anger	Joy	Pensiveness	Grief	Fear

Now let's explore them in a little more depth. Keep in mind that we'll be discussing the way food and nutrition fit into the overall Five Elements theory in Chapter 2. For now, you can see how the Chinese apply the cyclical nature of the seasons and the qualities of the natural elements to the human body.

The Fire Element is associated with summer. Its organs are the heart and the small intestine. In TCM, the heart is called the King of organs and is considered a yin organ. *The Yellow Emperor's Classic of Internal Medicine* states, "The heart commands all of the organs and viscera, houses the spirit, and controls the emotions." Physiologically, the heart controls the circulation and distribution of blood, and therefore all the other organs depend upon it for sustenance. It also influences thoughts and emotions. The small intestine is a yang organ. It is known as the Minister of Reception because it receives partially digested food from the stomach and spleen and further refines it. It also influences the function of the pituitary gland, whose secretions help to regulate growth, metabolism, and other endocrine functions.

The Earth Element is associated with late summer, a time between the intensity of summer and the decline of autumn. The yang stomach and the yin spleen-pancreas, which act together as one organ in TCM, are Earth organs. Called the Minister of the Mill, the stomach is responsible for providing the entire body with energy from the digestion of food. The spleen-pancreas, also known as the Minister of the Granary, provides the stomach and small intestine with enzymes necessary for digestion. It also regulates the quantity and quality of blood in circulation and controls fluid balance throughout the body.

The Metal Element, associated with fall, has the lungs as its yin organ and the large intestine as its yang organ. The lungs control breath and energy and work closely with the heart to circulate nourishment throughout the body. The large intestine, called the Minister of Transportation, controls the last part of the digestive process during which solid waste is formed and sent outward for excretion. By performing this function, the large intestine helps maintain the body's proper fluid balance and purity.

The Water Element, as its name suggests, has the kidney as its yin organ and the bladder as its yang organ. It is associated with winter. Known as the Minister of Power, the kidney represents the body's most important energy storage site. In addition to filtering waste products from the blood and moving them to the bladder for excretion, the kidneys also control sexual and reproductive functions and represent the body's prime source of sexual vitality. The bladder, also known as the Minister of the Reservoir, is responsible for storing and excreting urinary waste products. It also forms an important link to the autonomic nervous system, which helps to control relatively automatic functions like breathing and respiration.

The Wood Element is associated with spring and includes the liver (the General), a yin organ, and the gallbladder (the Honorable Minister) a yang organ. To find the underlying cause of disease, practitioners of Chinese medicine often look first to the liver, which is responsible for detoxifying, nourishing, replenishing, and storing blood. It acts to energize blood by releasing stored sugar, and it recombines amino acids derived from food to create the protein needed to grow and repair bodily tissues. Because the liver is linked to the peripheral nervous system, which regulates muscular activity and tension, a liver imbalance sometimes results in nervousness, rage, and anger. The gallbladder works with the lymphatic system to remove toxins from the muscles, thereby helping to soothe muscle aches and fatigue.

A Cycle of Balance

It's important to remember not simply the qualities that each of the Five Elements embodies, but also how one element relates to the others. Indeed, each of the Five Elements represents a stage of change, and each stage of change nourishes the next with the passage of qi. For example, the Fire element (summer) provides qi to the heart and small intestine, then passes it on to the Earth element (late summer), which nourishes the stomach and spleen. Earth (late summer) nourishes Metal (autumn). Metal (autumn) nourishes Water (winter), which then nourishes Wood (spring). This path of the qi throughout the body's parts is known as the Sheng Cycle.

At the same time, everything exists in balance, which means that there must be internal limits as well as releases. Fire controls Metal, and thus the heart and small intestine control or limit the energy within the lungs and large intestine. Because Earth controls Water, the stomach and spleen-pancreas check the energy flowing within the kidneys and bladder. Water controls Fire, and so the kidneys and bladder control the energy within the heart and small intestine. Wood controls Earth, thus the liver and gallbladder limit and regulate the energy flowing through the stomach and spleen-pancreas. This system of checks and balances is known as the Ke Cycle.

As you can see, although each organ in the body has its own unique structure, location, and physiologic activity, it is only when they all work together in balance and harmony that a human body is healthy. When something disrupts the balance of yin/yang or upsets the flow of qi, the Five Elements can no longer exist in their sublime equilibrium. In the next section, we'll show you what can occur inside and outside the body to disturb this equilibrium.

• *Patterns of Disharmony and Disease*

Illness in Chinese medicine is considered to be a state of imbalance in the body, an imbalance attributable to either external, internal, or neutral causes. External causes, called the Six Evils, originate outside the body. The internal causes, called the Seven Emotions, occur within the body itself. Neutral causes include lifestyle factors (diet and exercise habits) as well as what we think of as germs (viruses and bacteria) and injuries. Since neutral factors are those we in the West are most familiar with, let's take a look at the Chinese concept of external and internal causes of disease in more depth.

The Six Evils

The Six Evils are external forces in the universe that can invade the body and cause disease. The ancient Chinese recognized six different environmental conditions: wind, cold, heat, dampness, dryness, and fire. When these conditions invade the body, they may cause disease. The Six Evils also correspond to the Five Elements and seasons.

Evil	Element	Season	Organs	Emotion	Effects
Wind	Wood	Spring	Liver, gallbladder	Anger	Scatters, disperses
Heat	Fire	Summer	Heart, small intestine	Joy	Activates, ascends, warms
Damp	Earth	Late summer	Spleen, stomach	Pensiveness	Stagnates, sinks, condenses
Dry	Metal	Autumn	Lungs, large intestine	Grief	Shrinks, dehydrates
Cold	Water	Winter	Kidneys, bladder	Fear	Chills, depletes, exhausts
Fire	Exposure to any of the other five evils may give rise to fire, which intensifies symptoms and "burns out" affected organs and tissues.				

Each of the Six Evils influences the development of disease in a different way. Let's take them one by one:

Wind: Wind is a yang pathogen and related to spring within the Five Elements. Wind's nature is movement that rises and falls unpredictably and thus disturbs the location and direction of things. It has the effect of penetrating the exterior of the body and often combines with other external factors, like cold and heat, to invade the tissues. A common wind condition is the cold or flu: if qi is weak, then wind and cold can readily penetrate the surface of the body and invade the lungs. Wind can also be related to an internal disharmony, often involving the liver. *Internal liver wind* is the Chinese term for a condition that involves a serious disharmony and can result in stroke or Parkinson's disease.

Cold: Cold is associated with the season of winter and is considered a yin pathogen. If cold invades the body, you'll feel a chilly malaise, with headache and body aches and pains. Cold can affect not only the lungs, as described above, but also the stomach and spleen-pancreas, which can lead to vomiting and diarrhea. Internal cold usually results from a chronic deficient yang energy and can cause cold hands and feet and diarrhea, among other problems.

Dampness: Dampness, a yin pathogen, creates problems that are wet, heavy, and slow to clear up. When dampness invades the body, a person will experience symptoms of sluggishness and lethargy. The spleen-pancreas is especially vulnerable to dampness and when it is invaded by this pathogen, abdominal problems including diarrhea and cramping can occur. Arthritic conditions, too, are often related to dampness that invades the joints. Dampness is associated with late summer and Earth.

Dryness and Heat: Both dryness and heat are considered yang pathogens, one related to autumn and the other to summer. The symptoms of dry and heat diseases are similar: dry skin, parched lungs, exhaustion, headaches, and dehydration. The only distinction here is that dryness symptoms tend to be less severe than those of heat.

Fire: Fire evil is created when any of the seasonal energies becomes extreme over a long period of time. Fire evil works to "burn out" the affected organ's energy system. Its symptoms include fevers, inflammation, hyperactivity, and mental agitation. Fire conditions tend to be most associated with the liver, the stomach, and the lungs.

These six external causes of disharmony represent the environmental influences on our health. Our risk of exposure to them depends to some degree upon the climate in which we live as well as the strength of our qi at any given time. Part of that strength comes from how we feel inside, and how well we handle our emotional lives.

The Seven Emotions

In addition to the outside forces that may undermine one's health, Chinese medicine identifies seven internal conditions that can disrupt the body's flow of energy and yin/yang balance and harmony. In fact, unlike Western medicine, Chinese medicine considers extreme emotions to be as potentially pathogenic as any bacterium or virus. Within this context, there are seven different emotional avenues for disease: joy, anger, anxiety, pensiveness, grief, fear, and fright. When present in excess, each influences a specific organ in a particular way.

Joy: In Chinese medicine, joy refers not to a sense of happiness the way we think of it in the West, but to a state of overexcitement or agitation. Related to Fire, joy affects the heart, leading to feelings of nervousness, problems with insomnia, and heart palpitations.

Anger: This emotion, which may also involve feelings of resentment and frustration, gives rise to problems with the liver qi. Interestingly, the term *bilious* reflects the connection between anger and the liver: it means both "of a peevish ill-natured disposition" and "suffering from liver dysfunction." Stagnant liver qi often results in headaches and dizziness and, over the long term, in stomach and spleen-pancreas problems. Anger is associated with the Wood element.

Anxiety: As we in the West are slowly but surely beginning to understand, anxiety and stress are very harmful, impacting directly on the development of heart disease and hypertension. "Anxiety blocks energy and injures the lungs," states *The Yellow Emperor's Classic of Internal Medicine.* "It congests the breathing apparatus and suppresses respiration." Without proper breathing and circulation, qi cannot flow through the body properly and thus many organs and systems, including the cardiovascular system, begin to fail. Anxiety also affects the large intestine, causing gastrointestinal distress such as constipation and colitis.

Pensiveness: Excessive concentration, which we think of as chronic worry or obsessiveness, disrupts the yin spleen-pancreas and its yang counterpart, the stomach. As in the West, worry is seen in the East as a major cause of indigestion and other types of gastrointestinal distress, including ulcers.

Grief: The heart and lungs are the organs most affected by grief, sorrow, or chronic pessimism and negativity. When these emotions affect the heart and lungs—which are the wellspring from which energy and body fluids flow—they cause a depletion of qi throughout the body and thereby lower the body's defense against disease. Here, too, a similar connection between an emotion and a physical symptom is appreciated by the average American, if not officially recognized by the medical establishment: How often do we see a husband fall ill shortly after his wife passes away? How often do you fall ill under prolonged stress that overwhelms you or undermines your confidence?

Fear: More aptly described in this context as dread or gloom, fear affects kidney and bladder energy, causing problems in these organs. In fact, Chinese practitioners often relate children's bedwetting problems with childhood fears and nightmares.

Fright: Fright is a sudden, unexpected reaction that shocks the system. It causes energy to dissipate and injures the heart. If fright becomes chronic fear, it affects the kidney and bladder as well.

— ◄

Yin/yang, qi, the Five Elements, the Six Evils, and the Seven Emotions: Practitioners of Chinese medicine examine and evaluate all of these aspects of life and living during the diagnostic process.

• *Diagnosing the Chinese Way*

The first time you visit a healer who practices Chinese medicine, you may be surprised at the course the exam takes. Generally speaking, Chinese medicine provides no universal diagnostic criteria nor offers standard treatment plans. Instead, you'll be evaluated based on your own unique constitution, energy level, and symptoms. You'll notice, for instance, that you'll spend far more time than usual discussing your symptoms as well as aspects of your life and lifestyle that a Chinese healer may find relevant to your general health.

The physical examination consists of four different areas of exploration, called the four examinations. They are: looking, hearing and smelling, questioning, and touching. Let's take them one by one:

Looking: A practitioner relies first on a keen sense of observation. He or she will look at the way you move (a strong, lithe body is less likely to suffer from a deficient condition, for example), your general demeanor, the color and tone of your skin (dry skin suggests a blood deficiency and a red face indicates internal or external heat, for example), and the physical characteristics of your tongue.

As strange as it may seem to Westerners, Eastern practitioners believe that body disturbances are best reflected in the tongue. Indeed, the art of diagnosing disorders by observing changes in the tongue has been a primary aspect of Chinese medicine for centuries. Specifically, practitioners look at the shape of your tongue, its color, and its markings. They are able to discern even slight variations— variations not only unrecognizable to Westerners but sometimes even indescribable—and relate those variations to disorders. Here are the nearly two dozen tongue characteristics a practitioner considers:

Characteristic	Significance
Pale red tongue	Normal
Pale tongue	Deficient condition
Red tongue	Internal heat
Purple tongue	Stagnation of blood
Blue/black tongue	Internal cold
Thin tongue	Deficient condition
Swollen tongue	Internal damp
Stiff tongue	Internal wind
Quivering tongue	Spleen-pancreas deficiency
Short horizontal cracks	Spleen-pancreas deficiency
Toothmarks on sides	Spleen-pancreas deficiency
Shallow midline crack	Stomach deficiency
Long deep midline crack to tip	Heart deficiency or excess
Thin white coating	Normal
Thick white coating	Presence of disease
No coat	Yin deficiency
Medium white coat	Internal cold
Yellow coat	Internal heat
Slightly moist	Normal
Wet	Internal damp
Sticky	Phlegm
Dry	Internal heat

Hearing and Smelling: You might be surprised at the attention a practitioner of Chinese medicine pays to such matters as the tone of your voice (a loud, penetrating voice might indicate an excess condition, for instance) as well as how loudly or softly you breathe. A practitioner also will smell your breath and your body to gather further information: the presence of an unpleasant odor suggests the presence of heat, whereas no smell at all indicates cold.

Questioning: The practitioner will ask you lots of questions, such as how you tend to react to heat and cold, dampness and dryness, seasonal variations, and day-to-night changes in mood. Other questions might concern the frequency and qualities of your bowel movements, menstruation, and eating and drinking habits. The practitioner will also ask you about your symptoms, both the ones that brought you to him or her in the first place and those you might not have thought to mention. Your answers will give the practitioner an idea of what part of your system is out of balance and what kind of treatment you need to return it to a state of internal harmony.

Touching: The last step in the examination involves touching, or palpation, and the taking of your pulse. Through palpation, the practitioner measures the temperature of your skin, feels how moist or dry your skin is, and locates any tender or painful parts of your body. Pulse taking is considered one of the most important aspects of the diagnostic procedure in Chinese medicine. It involves recognizing about twenty-eight different qualities related to the pulse, which is taken at three different positions on both wrists.

Based on the information he or she collects during the examination, the practitioner evaluates the state of balance (or imbalance) in your body. Depending on where and in what way your body's natural state has been disrupted, the practitioner develops a treatment plan.

The Eight Indicators

The Eight Indicators are four sets of categories that help the practitioner interpret the data gathered by examination and thus reach a decision on treatment. These indicators determine the relative nature, quality, and location of qi within the body. Let's take them one by one:

Yin/Yang: Called the Commanders of the Eight Indicators, yin and yang represent the core of the diagnostic process. The practitioner first determines if the symptoms are more yin (chills, diarrhea, pallid complexion, chronic fatigue, etc.) or more yang (fever, constipation, sweating, and hypertension), then attempts to identify their nature (cold or hot), find their location (internal or external), and determine their effect on the body (causing a deficiency or an excess).

Cold (Yin)/Heat (Yang): Cold and hot indicate the basic nature of the disease as reflected by its symptoms—high or low temperature, flushed or pale complexion, hard or soft stools, etc. Cold symptoms include depressed metabolic activity, an aversion to cold, low body temperature, loose stools, profuse and light-colored urine, lassitude and indifference. Heat symptoms include an overactive metabolism, aversion to heat, high body temperature, constipation, scant and dark-colored urine, nervousness and emotional instability.

Interior/Exterior: The practitioner tries to find where the disease is located and in what direction it is moving. If symptoms are moving toward the organs, it indicates that the disease is getting worse, whereas if they seem to be moving outward, the patient's condition is improving.

Deficiency/Excess: This set of indicators refers to the degree to which an ailment has depleted (indicating deficiency) or overstimulated (indicating excess) the organs, fluids, and energies of the body.

It should be noted that the Eight Indicators are not considered separate, discrete categories. Instead, they often exist in combinations of patterns. For example, someone might have symptoms that indicate an invasion of wind cold, which is an exterior/excess pattern with cold predominating. If this condition is not treated, it may turn to a wind heat problem (yin becoming yang), which is an exterior/excess pattern with heat predominating.

Once the practitioner identifies the pattern of disharmony that has caused your symptoms, he or she will decide upon a course of treatment. As you might imagine, the nature of the pattern may shift as treatment progresses, as yin becomes yang. Most likely, treatment will consist of a combination of acupuncture, herbal medicine, and nutritional advice.

• *Healing in the Chinese Tradition*

If you're like most of your Western compatriots, you're used to going to the doctor whenever you have symptoms that make you feel uncomfortable. The doctor examines you, performs certain laboratory tests, then diagnoses a specific condition that he or she attempts to resolve with a standard treatment, usually involving medication or surgery or both. For a vast majority of illnesses, however, especially those of a chronic nature like heart disease, arthritis, allergies, and gastritis, these solutions can be dissatisfying: either the side effects from medication or surgery are too great to bear, or the underlying causes of the condition are never addressed, and so fester and persist no matter what the treatment. In Eastern medicine, however, alleviating symptoms is secondary to addressing the root of the problem—the imbalances within the body.

Acupuncture and Acupressure

One key to proper health is keeping qi flowing properly through the body. Acupuncture and its massage-related cousin, acupressure, are designed to release qi that has become blocked or stagnant. Throughout the body, there are over one thousand *acupoints,* areas that can be stimulated to enhance the flow of qi. When a trained professional inserts special needles into these points, they help to correct the flow of energy and thus work to restore health. The exact point of insertion depends on the site of the disharmony and the way in which the practitioner wishes to influence the qi. You shouldn't feel any pain when he or she inserts the needle, although you may feel a mild pinprick as the needle pierces the skin.

Acupuncture needles may be inserted to a depth of about ¼ inch to 2 inches or more, depending on a variety of factors, including your size and the part of the body concerned. Needles are left in place for a few seconds or up to an hour; the average treatment time being about twenty minutes. Along with needles, moxibustion is often used to warm and tone the body's qi. Special herbs called moxa, derived from the herb mugwort, are heated and placed directly above a specific acupoint.

Some historians believe that the Chinese developed the technique of moxibustion even before they invented acupuncture. Northern Chinese, who huddled around campfires to warm themselves, learned to light twigs, grasses, and leaves, then place the hot mixture on areas of the body experiencing pain. Today, practitioners light tightly wrapped leaves of the moxa plant, then hold the glowing end close to the vital point they want to treat. The energy of the burning herb penetrates through the surface, into the point, and travels to the targeted organs and tissues.

As its name implies, acupressure massage involves physical manipulation of acupoints with the fingers and palms of the practitioner's hands.

Herbal Medicine

The use of herbs is an essential part of traditional Chinese medicine. Herbs help to reorganize the body constituents (qi, blood, and body fluids) within the meridians and organs, as well as help the body adjust to the impact of any external evils like wind, cold, or dampness.

In general, Chinese herbal medicine involves using multiple herbs in combinations that have specific effects. In addition to these combinations, practitioners can prescribe single herbs to alleviate particular symptoms. For instance, a diuretic herb, like the fungus *Poria cocos,* may be prescribed to someone who has high blood pressure related to water retention. Herbs are also classified according to the Five Elements theory, with specific flavors and qualities that allow the practitioner to match them to an illness.

Herbs contain a large number of naturally occurring substances that work to alter the body's chemistry in order to return it to its natural state of health. Unlike purified drugs, however, plants and other organic materials contain a wide variety of substances and, hence, less of any one particular active alkaloid. This attribute makes herbs far less potentially toxic to the body than most pharmaceutical products.

Another benefit of natural herbs is that they tend to contain combinations of substances that work together to restore balance to the body with a minimum of side effects. The plant meadowsweet is a good example: it contains compounds similar to those in aspirin that act as anti-inflammatories. These compounds, called salicylates, often irritate the stomach lining. Unlike commercially prepared aspirin, however, meadowsweet also contains substances that soothe the gastric lining and reduce stomach acidity, thus providing relief from pain while protecting the stomach from irritation.

Herbs of all types are available in many forms including:

Raw: Eating herbs in their fresh state is the most ancient method of taking them and, depending on the herb, the most efficient way of using herbs as medicine.

Whole: Plants or plant parts are dried and either cut or powdered to be used as teas or as cooking herbs. You'll see how the Chinese use herbs in cooking in Part III.

Capsules and Tablets: Increasingly popular with consumers, capsules and tablets allow patients to consume herbs quickly and without tasting those that are strong or bitter.

Extracts and Tinctures: Extracts and tinctures are made by grinding the roots, leaves, and/or flowers of an herb and immersing them in a solution of alcohol and water for a period of time; the alcohol works both to extract the maximum amount of active ingredients from the herb and to preserve those elements.

Poultices and Ointments: Ground herbs form the base of external applications that you can place directly on your skin. Poultices are hot packs applied to the skin. They are made by mixing ground herbs with hot water, placing them in a muslin bag, and then applying them to the area suggested by the practitioner. An ointment is a cream or salve with an herbal base that you can buy in health food stores or order through your practitioner.

As you can see, Chinese herbal medicine is a complex and multilayered science. Only a small part of that science involves using herbs as medicine in cooking, as you'll see in Chapter 2. If you're interested in further exploring this aspect of Chinese herbal medicine, see the Resource Guide for organizations to contact and books to read for more information.

Qi-gong

A third form of therapy in Chinese medicine is qi-gong, which literally translates as "energy exercises." Qi-gong builds qi and helps move it freely around the body. There are several different types of qi-gong. Some exercises are similar to calisthenics or isometric movements; others are meditative stances; still others involve the stimulation of acupressure points with massage. Breathing exercises are designed to bring the body into a state of relaxation and harmony. All qi-gong exercises attempt to cultivate inner strength, calm the mind, and help maintain or restore the body's natural state of internal balance and harmony.

Nutrition

As discussed, each type of food—from fruits and vegetables to game and fish to herbs and spices—has its own specific quality and action on the body. After diagnosing your condition, a practitioner will work with you to create an eating plan that stresses the foods that will help bring your body back into balance and keep it there. In Chapter 2, you'll learn more about nutrition and health from both a Western and an Eastern perspective.

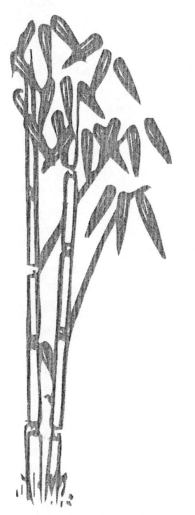

CHAPTER TWO

The Healing Properties of Food

"**F**OOD IS MEDICINE AND medicine is food." So states a well-known Chinese proverb that aptly reflects the way the Chinese view and apply the principles of nutrition. We here in the West have a couple adages of our own relating food to health, including "You are what you eat" and "Thy food be thy medicine." In the past few decades, people all over the world have come to a greater understanding of nutrition and its importance to their physical and mental well-being. In this chapter you'll discover the role food plays in traditional Chinese medicine. You'll also receive a miniprimer on Western concepts of nutrition so that by the time you delve into healing with nutrition in Part II, you'll have a basic East/West understanding of how eating can be an important element in attaining and maintaining health.

As you might suspect after reading Chapter 1, Western and Eastern branches of medicine offer quite different perspectives on the role of diet in health and healing. Here in the West, we tend to focus on food primarily for the way it impacts upon our weight (its calorie count and fat content) or for its biochemical constituents (the amount and type of vitamins, minerals, protein, fiber, and other compounds it contains). In recent years, we've discovered the vital role those components play in both keeping us healthy and healing us once an illness develops. Later in the chapter, we discuss the principles of a healthy diet based on these concepts.

Nutrition also plays an important role in Chinese medicine. It is not merely an afterthought as it so often seems here in the West. The Chinese see food as an integral part of nature. Each food has qualities of yin/yang and the Five Elements that affect our bodies in an intimate and essential way. The theory goes that in order to stay healthy, we need to eat foods in specific combinations and amounts that depend upon our particular body type, constitution, and lifestyle.

When prescribing treatment for a specific pattern of disharmony, a practitioner selects foods based on their particular qualities as they apply to these theories. If you complain of feeling chilly and congested, for instance, your doctor of Chinese medicine might well prescribe foods that can warm you and soothe your internal dryness. If you feel hot and constipated, on the other hand, your doctor will probably prescribe cooling foods to alleviate the internal heat causing your symptoms. Let's take a closer look at these aspects of nutrition from an Eastern perspective.

• *Nutrition from the East*

Balance and moderation are the keys to healthy eating, in the East and in the West. However, as is true for so many aspects of the philosophy of traditional Chinese medicine, the principles of diet and nutrition remain highly individualized. As discussed, it is impossible to recommend specific healthy foods for the population in general. You—as a unique person with your own physiology, body type, metabolism, emotional makeup, and lifestyle—have your own unique formula for attaining and maintaining health.

However, there are some general guidelines for creating a balanced and healthy eating plan based on TCM. The first thing to remember is that the stomach and the spleen-pancreas are the two main organs of digestion. Providing them with the right amount and type of food is crucial to maintaining health. For instance, cold food puts a strain on the stomach and too much cold food slows down digestion and chills the body. That's why you should moderate the amount of raw vegetables or chilled juices you eat and drink. Food that is indigestible because it is of poor quality or because you've failed to chew it well also puts a strain on the stomach. Choosing fresh foods then obviously becomes another important element of healthy eating. So, too, is eating slowly and chewing carefully.

Once food has been digested by the stomach, it moves to the spleen-pancreas, where it undergoes another set of transformations to become one of the body's vital substances. If the spleen-pancreas functions poorly or if we eat the wrong foods, we simply will not have the raw material we need to live well. In Part II, you'll probably notice how many conditions apparently unrelated to the digestive system are alleviated by bolstering the stomach and spleen-pancreas.

Although each individual has a different set of nutritional requirements, the Chinese do have some general recommendations as to what raw material your body needs, and in what proportion. Later in the chapter, we outline the American idea of a balanced diet as prescribed by the Food Pyramid devised by the American Dietetic Association. Like the Food Pyramid plan, in a healthy Chinese diet complex carbohydrates, like rice, fruits, and vegetables, are the mainstay, and the amounts of protein, dairy, fat, and sugar are limited. But the Chinese look at diet and its role in health and disease quite differently than we do in the West.

The Yin and Yang of Food

As you may remember from Chapter 1, yin and yang are two dynamic energies, two polar forces that together maintain balance and harmony throughout the entire universe and within each individual human body. Every herb, vegetable, meat, fish, grain, and dairy product has its own relationship to yin and yang. It is a relationship that changes depending upon any number of factors, including the season in which you eat it and the way you prepare it. Yin foods are more cooling, for instance, which means that raw vegetables are generally considered to have more yin energy than cooked vegetables, which have been heated.

Some other examples of yin/yang relationships to specific foods follow:

Yin Foods	Yang Foods
Raw fruits	Dried and stewed fruits
Raw vegetables	Cooked vegetables
Tofu	Cabbage
Seaweed	Tomato sauce
Bulgar	Root vegetables
Rice	Lentils, kidney beans
Milk, yogurt	Potatoes
Raw fish	Nuts, seeds
	Beef, lamb, chicken, cooked fish

Yin foods tend to have a cooling, calming effect on human energy, while yang foods are warming and stimulating. When a practitioner prescribes food to help restore balance, he or she looks first to the yin/yang quality of a symptom: fever, for instance, is a yang condition and so should be treated by eating cooling yin foods, whereas constipation is a yin condition that you might want to treat by eating warming yang foods.

In addition to their yin/yang qualities, foods also have what are known as *flavors* that further influence the way the body functions.

Yang foods, for instance, have sweet pungent flavors that tend to energize the body, while yin foods have salty, bitter, or sour flavors that help to build the blood and other body fluids.

The Five Flavors of Foods

Pungent, sweet, sour, bitter, salty: these are the Five Flavors that foods have within the Chinese philosophy of medicine and healing. Each different flavor has a specific effect on our organs, and each food has a different effect on the body depending on its flavor. Although some flavors attributed to foods seem obvious—seafood is salty, for example—others correspond less clearly to what we in the West think of as flavor. Beef, for instance, is considered a sweet food and asparagus a pungent one, tastes most Westerners would be unlikely to associate with these particular foods. In addition, some foods have more than one associated taste: pork is considered a sweet and salty food, leeks are considered sour and pungent, yogurt sour and sweet, and papaya bitter and sweet.

Let's see how each flavor acts on the body:

Pungent: Pungent, or acrid, foods (which have a yang energy) help to induce perspiration, disperse mucus, and promote energy circulation. They enter the lungs to clear them of mucus, improve digestive activity, and stimulate blood circulation. The pungent flavor is related to the spring season. Some pungent foods are ginger, green onion, taro, turnip, kohlrabi, and peppermint.

Sweet: Sweet foods also have a yang energy, but work to slow down the progression of some symptoms and neutralize the toxic effects of other foods. Sweet foods strengthen the spleen-pancreas and soothe the liver. They work best during the late summer, which is the juncture between summer and fall, what Westerners might identify as August and September. They moisten dry conditions of the lungs and help calm emotional distress. Sweet foods include sweet rice, sweet potato, eggplant, carrots, molasses, walnuts, honey, sugar, watermelon, chestnuts, bananas, and beef.

Sour: Sour foods like lemon, plum, pear, and mango work to obstruct bodily functions, which make them helpful in alleviating diarrhea, excessive perspiration, and hemorrhoids, among other conditions. Sour foods are most active in the liver, where they counteract the effects of rich, greasy food. Sour foods are related to the fall season.

Bitter: Bitter foods have a yin, cooling effect on the body. They are helpful in reducing inflammation and alleviating infections. They also help to lower blood pressure. Bitter foods are most effective in the fall and winter months. Lettuce, radish, alfalfa, romaine lettuce, scallion, and vinegar are among those foods considered bitter.

Salty: Like bitter foods, salty foods are considered to have yin, cooling effects on the body. They work to moisten dry conditions, improve digestion, detoxify the body, and can purge the bowels and promote urination. The cooling nature of the salty flavor relates to the colder seasons and climates; therefore they should be used more in the fall and winter than at other times of the year.

After a practitioner of Chinese medicine evaluates your condition by the methods described in Chapter 1, he or she will devise a treatment plan that includes dietary prescriptions aimed at restoring yin/yang balance and a free-flowing qi within your body. By understanding the flavor, nature, and action of each food, the practitioner is able to create an eating plan that's just right for your particular body chemistry and current imbalance. That's why it's very important for you to visit a qualified practitioner of Chinese medicine before you attempt to treat any illness or condition with nutrition alone. Only by doing so will you be sure to effectively address your needs with the foods you eat.

Now that you see how food fits into the general TCM philosophy, let's take a look at each type and its action in the body:

Water

Although we don't often see water listed as a nutrient, it is in fact the most abundant nutrient in the body, comprising about two thirds of the body's mass. As we'll discuss later, Western medicine suggests drinking at least 64 ounces of water every day. According to the principles of TCM, however, there is no set prescription for the amount of water you should drink. In fact, an old Zen maxim states the equation quite simply: "Eat when hungry, drink when thirsty." However, since many of us lose touch with our body's true needs, a few general suggestions can be made. On average, you'll need to drink *less* water if you are sedentary, eat plenty of fresh fruits and vegetables (which are often more than 90 percent water), have a cold or deficient condition as diagnosed by a practitioner of Chinese medicine, and/or live in a cold or damp climate. You'll need to drink comparatively more water if you partake in strenuous exercise, consume a lot of meat, eggs, and/or salty food, suffer from fever or other heat conditions, and/or live in a dry, hot, or windy climate.

Grains

Grains should make up about 40 to 60 percent of your diet. The Chinese consider rice to be the most nourishing grain because it is neither too hot nor too cold. It also works to clear away dampness, one of the most pervasive of the Six Evils you read about in Chapter 1. Dampness forms when body fluids and qi do not move through the body properly. Bloating, lethargy, and poor concentration often result from dampness, as do some common chronic illnesses like arthritis, allergies, and constipation.

Other grains work in different ways on the body. A practitioner of Chinese medicine is likely to suggest the types of grains you should eat based on an evaluation of your particular body type, constitution, and your current condition. Here are some suggestions:

Excess Condition: If you are a strong, hearty person with a reddish complexion, you might want to stick with grains that work to reduce excess, such as rye and wild rice.

Deficient Condition: If you feel weak and have low energy, almost any grain will help restore your balance, including rice, wheat, and cooked oats.

Heat Condition: If you often feel thirst, frequently run fevers, and have a reddish complexion, cooling grains are best for you. Millet, wheat, wild rice, and whole barley are some to try.

Cold Condition: Warming grains like oats, sweet rice, and basmati rice are right for you if you often crave hot food and beverages, have a pale complexion, and often feel cold.

Damp Condition: If you often feel sluggish and have swelling, obesity, and/or chronic mucus problems, you'll probably want to eat grains that reduce dampness. Buckwheat, corn, rye, wild rice, and dry roasted oats are best for you in that case.

Dry Condition: If you have a tendency to be underweight and have dry skin, you might be well served by adding wheat, rice, sweet rice (made by adding sugar, fruit, or other sweetener to the cooking process), and barley to your diet.

Legumes

Legumes are sources of protein and roughage and should be included in your diet at least 2–3 times a week. Included in this category are lentils, kidney beans, chickpeas, and bean curd. As a rule, legumes tend to bring back into balance excess symptoms, such as swelling, redness, and a tendency to be overweight, but each type of legume works on a different part of the body. Red legumes, such as red lentils and kidney beans, influence the heart and small intestines; yellow legumes, such as garbanzo beans and soybeans, influence the spleen-pancreas and stomach; white legumes, such as lima beans and navy beans, influence the lungs and large intestine; dark brown legumes, such as black beans and brown lentils, influence the kidneys and bladder; and green legumes, such as green peas and green beans, influence the liver and gallbladder.

Keep in mind that some people find legumes difficult to digest. It's important to chew them thoroughly and limit the amount you eat—just a few tablespoons have high nutritional and healing value. They combine best with green or nonstarchy vegetables. Grains and beans make a particularly potent combination in both Eastern and Western cooking, since they provide all the essential amino acids in one complete meal.

Fruits and Vegetables

Fresh fruits and vegetables should make up about 20 to 30 percent of your diet. If possible, choose organic produce, which is higher in vitamins and minerals and greatly reduces your exposure to pesticides and other harmful chemicals. The Chinese recommend that you cook your vegetables before you eat them because cooked vegetables are more easily digested and assimilated by the body than raw vegetables.

The healing properties of vegetables and fruits depend very much on their individual flavors and properties. Most fruits have a sweet flavor and cooling nature that helps to balance any rich foods you might eat. They act to stimulate the liver and spleen-pancreas to offer a natural laxative effect. Certain other fruits, including blackberries, plums, and pineapple are sour and constricting, and are often prescribed to treat diarrhea. Here are some more examples of fruits and the way they act in the body:

Fruit	Flavor	Nature	Good for
Apricot	Sweet-sour	Neutral	Lung conditions
Banana	Sweet	Cool	Lubricating organs
Kumquat	Pungent	Warm	Eliminating mucus
Lemon/lime	Sour	Cool	Fighting infections
Orange	Sweet-sour	Cool	Weak digestion
Pineapple	Sweet-sour	Neutral	Diarrhea
Raspberry	Sweet-sour	Neutral	Liver and kidneys

When it comes to vegetables, the healing properties are even more specific to each vegetable. Asparagus, for instance, is bitter-pungent, slightly warming, and helps to eliminate water through the kidneys. However, another dark green vegetable, broccoli, is slightly bitter and cooling—but also works as a diuretic. Lets take a look at some more examples:

Fruit	Flavor	Nature	Good for
Beet	Sweet	Neutral	Heart and blood
Cabbage	Sweet-pungent	Warming	Digestion
Carrot	Sweet	Neutral	Lungs, liver, spleen
Celery	Sweet-bitter	Cool	Reducing heat
Eggplant	Sweet	Cool	Reducing bleeding
Garlic	Pungent	Warm	Expelling cold
Kale	Sweet-bitter-pungent	Warm	Lung congestion
Lettuce	Bitter-sweet	Cool	Drying damp
Mushroom	Sweet	Cool	Reducing mucus
Potato	Sweet	Neutral	Digestion
Tomato	Sweet-sour	Cool	Relieving dryness
Yam	Sweet	Cool	Promoting qi

Meat and Dairy

The Chinese consider meat, poultry, seafood, and dairy foods to be highly nutritious and very rich foods. Therefore, they eat only relatively small quantities of them at each meal. In a traditional Chinese diet, these foods make up only about 10 to 15 percent of the foods eaten daily.

Dairy products supply protein and vitamin B_{12} which can be especially helpful to vegetarians and people with deficient conditions. According to Chinese medicine, milk builds qi vitality and tonifies (or strengthens) the yin organs and body fluids. Dairy consumption, therefore, benefits thin and weak people with a tendency toward dryness. However, dairy foods can cause problems for some people because they can be mucus-producing and may be loaded with fat.

Eggs are another source of protein used quite often by the Chinese. Eggs are considered to have a neutral nature and a sweet flavor that nourishes yin. They have an "ascending direction," which means that they act to move energy and fluids higher in the body. (In Parts II and III, you'll see how helpful eggs can be when it comes to alleviating diarrhea and other "descending" conditions.)

When it comes to meat, poultry, and fish, the Five Elements structure establishes a relationship between specific body organs and corresponding animal products. The liver benefits from poultry, the heart from mutton and lamb, the spleen-pancreas from beef and veal, and the lung from fish. Therefore, if your practitioner diagnoses a weakness in your liver energy, for instance, he or she will likely recommend that you eat more chicken or duck. A weakness in the spleen-pancreas calls for more beef; in the lung, more fish; in the heart, more veal and mutton. In addition, each type of protein has a different flavor and thus a different action on the body. Clams, for instance, have a cooling nature, are salty, and help moisten dryness and nurture yin, while shrimp are warming and sweet and enhance yang. You'll see how each type of food helps restore specific imbalances in Parts II and III.

Fat

As for fat, the Chinese believe, as do Westerners, that fat should be used sparingly because it may cause an unhealthy weight gain and other medical problems. However, according to Chinese medical principles, fat is an important constituent in the diet. Fat bolsters yin, helps build body tissues, and enhances fluid metabolism. In China, people traditionally use roasted sesame oil and peanut oil for cooking and making condiments. These oils are natural and nonhydrogenated, and thus contain the important nutrients called *essential fatty acids.* By replacing fats with lowfat products in which natural fats have been replaced by hydrogenated vegetable oils, as we do so often here in the West, we deprive our bodies of the raw materials they need to function.

In Chapter 3, you'll see how the Chinese prepare meals using a variety of different ingredients and cooking methods to attain balance during times of general health. When it comes to healing, however, the principles of Chinese medicine involve choosing what you eat with attention to your body's individual needs and any imbalances that exist. You'll see more of what that means to your health in Part II.

• *A Western Nutritional Guide*

As you can see, traditional Chinese medicine looks at food and how it benefits the human body in a very different way than does modern Western medicine. Here in the West, we rarely consider how the temperature of the food we eat might affect our health, or how the seasons change the effects of food on the body. Instead, we concentrate on calories, fat grams, and percentages of Recommended Daily Allowances of vitamins and minerals.

For much of the twentieth century, Americans have consumed a diet very high in saturated fat, sugar, and protein. Many nutritionists believe that this diet is largely responsible for our most pressing health problems, including our high rates of heart disease, hypertension, diabetes, and cancer. Fortunately, more and more Americans are reexamining their eating habits and working to establish a healthy approach to food and nutrition. To help you get started thinking about your diet from a Western perspective, we've developed this miniguide to proper nutrition.

The human body requires about forty different types of "raw materials" in order to carry out its functions and maintain its health. These include oxygen, water, complex carbohydrates, vitamins and minerals, proteins, and fat. Your body receives oxygen from the air you breathe; without it, you couldn't survive for more than a few minutes. Although most of us take oxygen for granted, study after study proves that the more oxygen you supply to your body's cells—by breathing deeply and circulating more oxygen-rich blood during exercise—the better.

Water, which is found in most everything we eat and drink, is another substance we tend to take for granted. Water regulates body temperature, circulation, and excretion, and aids in digestion. It bathes virtually all of our cells in moisture. Nevertheless, few of us drink the 64 ounces (eight glasses) of water our body needs every day to stay healthy.

We attain the other thirty-eight or so essential nutrients in the food we eat. What we call a balanced diet is one that contains the appropriate amount—not too little and not too much—of certain foods that contain those nutrients on a daily basis. In addition, a balanced diet involves providing the right amount of calories—the energy value of food—to maintain proper body weight. (A calorie represents the amount of energy the body would need to burn in order to use up that bit of food; any excess energy is stored as fat.)

Most of us grew up with the idea that a balanced diet included equal amounts of four food groups: dairy, grains, meats, and fruits/vegetables. Several years ago, the American Dietetic Association developed a new way of looking at our daily diet. Called the Food Pyramid, it organizes food types into a pyramid of multisized compartments. Each compartment represents a type of food and the proportion of the daily diet it should comprise. Before we look at those categories, let's discuss five substances found in those foods that are the subject of much scrutiny when it comes to creating a healthy diet: dietary fiber, vitamins, minerals, phytochemicals, and cholesterol.

Dietary Fiber

Also called roughage, dietary fiber is a group of widely varied complex carbohydrates found in whole grains, fruits, and vegetables. Fiber is divided into two basic types—soluble and insoluble—and five major forms, cellulose, hemicellulose, lignin, pectin, and gums. Each type of plant food differs in the type and amount of fiber it contains.

Because the digestive process does not break down dietary fiber, fiber does not provide any energy to the body. Instead, it enters the large intestine more or less intact. In doing so, it helps to promote more efficient elimination by increasing stool bulk, and thus may alleviate some digestive disorders, particularly constipation.

Fiber is also known to protect against colon cancer (which is the second most common form of cancer in the United States), by helping keep the digestive system clean and clear. Soluble fiber also helps to reduce the amount of dietary cholesterol and glucose that enters the bloodstream, thus reducing the risk of heart disease and diabetes.

Vitamins, Minerals, and Phytochemicals

Vitamins are organic substances found in plants and animals. Generally speaking, the body cannot manufacture vitamins and so we must obtain them through our diet or the use of supplements. There are about fourteen vitamins considered vital to life, and several other nutrients whose roles are just beginning to be recognized.

Minerals, on the other hand, are inorganic substances that are basic constituents of the earth's crust. We get minerals by eating fruits, grains, and vegetables that have absorbed them from soil and groundwater. Of the more than sixty different minerals in the body, twenty-two are considered essential. Seven of these, including calcium, chloride, magnesium, phosphorus, potassium, sodium, and sulfur, are considered major minerals. Others, called trace minerals, are found in tiny amounts in the body, but their small quantities belie their importance.

Among the most important categories of vitamins and minerals are the antioxidants. Antioxidants such as vitamins C and E and beta-carotene have the ability to destroy certain harmful molecules in the body called free radicals, which can damage tissues. Free radical damage is linked to myriad diseases, including arthritis, cancer, and heart disease. A mineral called selenium is also considered an antioxidant, because it helps a powerful enzyme called glutathione peroxidase to do its job in the body—which is to render harmless certain free radicals called oxidized lipids. Zinc, another essential mineral, helps the body absorb and use antioxidants.

Phytochemicals are a recently recognized group of antioxidants related to vitamins and minerals; they are found in fruits and vegetables. There are literally thousands of phytochemicals, each of which appears to play a role in preventing cancer from taking hold in the body. One phytochemical compound, called sulforaphane, is found in broccoli, cauliflower, kale, and other cruciferous vegetables, as well as strawberries, raspberries, and grapes. Sulforaphane may protect us against breast and other cancers. Another, called phenethyl isothiocyanate (PEITC), appears to guard against lung cancer by essentially binding to carcinogens before they can reach healthy human cells. We obtain PEITC by eating turnips and cabbage. Genistein, found in soybeans, has been shown to prevent the growth of prostate tumors.

Cholesterol

A substance related to fat, cholesterol is perhaps the most infamous of all dietary substances, thanks in large part to the suspected role it plays in the development of heart disease. It is important to gain a deeper understanding of the role cholesterol plays in our health and in the development of disease.

Cholesterol is a lipid essential for a number of vital processes, including nerve function, cell repair and reproduction, and the formation of various hormones, including estrogen, testosterone, and the stress hormone cortisol. Because it is so important to the body, the liver works very hard to create all the cholesterol we need to survive. In fact, the liver produces about 3,000 milligrams of new cholesterol every twenty-four hours, a quantity equivalent to the amount contained in ten eggs.

And there's the rub when it comes to maintaining health: The body manufactures *all* the cholesterol it needs. Any cholesterol you consume is "extra" and can lead to health problems if there is enough of it circulating in the bloodstream. In addition, cholesterol-rich foods are frequently high in saturated fats (discussed below) and are often fried, leading to the conversion of the cholesterol to an activated and quite dangerous form.

Cholesterol travels through the bloodstream by combining with other lipids and certain proteins. When combined, these substances are called lipoproteins. One type of lipoprotein, called high-density lipoprotein (HDL), is beneficial to the body because it carries cholesterol away from the cells back to the liver, which processes it for elimination. You might know HDL-cholesterol as the "good" cholesterol.

Another type of lipoprotein is harmful to the body. Called low-density lipoprotein or LDL, this substance carries about two thirds of circulating cholesterol to the cells. This is often the "fat" we speak of when referring to the plaque that builds up and causes atherosclerosis or hardening of the arteries. Research indicates that LDL-cholesterol may become harmful only after it combines with oxygen. Oxidation occurs through a complicated chemical reaction in the body, a process that you may be able to prevent—or at least limit—by eating plenty of fruits and vegetables rich in B vitamins.

In foods, cholesterol is found primarily in animal products such as meats and dairy products, which also tend to be high in fat and calories. In addition, cooking foods in a way that exposes them to oxygen and/or raises their temperature to high levels may increase the amount of harmful cholesterol that eventually reaches your bloodstream. For instance, hard- or soft-boiled and poached eggs do not appear to raise cholesterol levels in most individuals, while scrambled or fried eggs often significantly raise levels of LDL. How much "bad" cholesterol you have circulating in your bloodstream is also directly related to how much fat you eat. In fact, cholesterol is only one of several different forms of fatlike substances that may act in a harmful way in the body.

At the same time, however, it is important to recognize that not all fat is bad fat. The fact remains that we need to consume a little fat—about the equivalent of one tablespoon every day—in order to survive. Fats perform several vital functions in the body. They store energy, help maintain healthy skin and hair, and carry fat-soluble vitamins (A, D, E, and K) through the bloodstream. They also provide the body with substances called essential fatty acids, which are the raw materials for several hormonelike compounds which help regulate blood pressure, the process of inflammation, and other body functions.

There are three major types of fats—saturate, monosaturate, and polyunsaturate—that are found in varying amounts in all foods that contain fat. It helps to know what kind of fat you're eating, because different fats affect your health (specifically the amount of "bad" cholesterol you have in your bloodstream).

Saturated fats are found in hydrogenated vegetable shortenings and in animal products such as whole milk, some cheeses, butter, meat, and cream. One way to recognize a saturated fat is that it is solid at room temperature. Processed peanut butter and margarine are two examples. Saturated fats are the fats to avoid; they raise the levels of cholesterol in the blood by 5 to 10 percent.

Monosaturated fats, like peanut oil and olive oil, remain liquid at room temperature. These fats may work to lower serum LDL levels. Olive oil, in particular, may lower LDL while keeping HDL levels the same, a net benefit to the body.

Unsaturated fats, also called *polyunsaturated fats,* consist of liquid vegetable oils, like sunflower, corn, soybean, and sesame. Important dietary unsaturated fats also come from plants and fish. Not only do these fats lower the amount of cholesterol in the body, those found in fish oil also contain the fatty acid called omega-3, which, as discussed above, have numerous health benefits.

According to the Pyramid Plan, you should try to limit your daily fat intake to 10 to 20 percent of your daily caloric intake. If you eat 2,000 calories a day, only 200 to 400 of those calories should consist of calories derived from fat. (200 calories equals about 21 grams of fat.) Stay away from fat from animal sources such as whole milk, cheese, fatty meats, and poultry, which are more likely to contain saturated fats. Eat more fatty, cold water fish such as salmon, mackerel, halibut, tuna, and sardines, which contain omega-3 fatty acids.

— —

From the East or from the West, the goal of nutrition remains the same: to provide your body—with its own unique attributes and qualities—with the ingredients it needs to remain healthy and balanced. Although the methods of achieving these goals may be quite different, there are some general prescriptions both cultures would agree upon:

Try to include more high-protein plant foods like grains, legumes, nuts, and seeds in your diet.

Buy and prepare seasonal foods. Vegetables and fruits grown out of season often have to be induced to grow with chemicals and artificial light, which may have negative health effects.

Avoid food additives and preservatives like aspartame, Red Dye #2, monosodium glutamate, nitrates, and sulfur dioxide found in most processed foods. Eat more fresh, whole foods.

Read food labels carefully—even if you're following a diet largely based on TCM tenets. It's important for you to remain aware of the quantities of essential nutrients, fat, and additives in the foods you eat.

Eat a variety of food to keep your taste buds satisfied, your body in balance, and your soul at peace.

Now that you've learned something about nutrition and its role in keeping us healthy and strong, it's time to look at how food can help heal the body once an internal imbalance occurs.

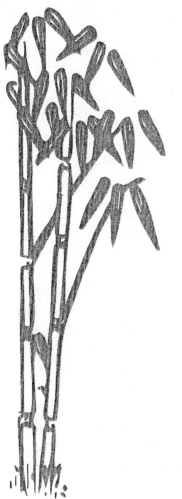

CHAPTER THREE

Preparing Your Kitchen

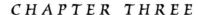

WHAT MAKES CHINESE cooking both delicious and healthy? One feature is the technique of stir-frying (described later in this chapter), which cooks meats and vegetables to a tender crispness with very little fat. Another factor is its rich flavors and textures, derived from the wide variety of vegetables and fruits, herbs, and spices used in each dish. Although the list of ingredients might seem exotic to you at first, or the cooking techniques and equipment a little unfamiliar, it won't be long before you'll feel perfectly comfortable preparing food the Chinese way.

• *Eating the Chinese Way*

If you like, you cannot only prepare and eat traditional Chinese food but you can also serve it in a traditional Chinese manner. Just follow these simple suggestions to attain a more Asian atmosphere:

Planning the Meal: While meals in the United States tend to revolve around one main dish of chicken, fish, or meat accompanied by a vegetable and a starch, a traditional Chinese meal focuses on rice or another grain surrounded by several meat and vegetable dishes. The number of dishes accompanying the rice depends on the number of people dining: generally speaking, a family of six may serve three or four dishes at dinner, two or three at lunch. Of course, if you're preparing a meal in order to solve a medicinal problem, it's important to choose dishes that attempt to restore the same type of imbalance—dishes that feature mostly cooling foods if you suffer from excess heat, for instance.

Setting the Table: Chinese meals are communal affairs with all dishes shared among guests. That's why, if possible, you should serve your meals at a round table that allows dishes—and conversation—to pass among diners with ease. Each place setting includes one rice bowl, a matching saucer (to hold the food passed from the communal dishes), and a pair of chopsticks. Place the chopsticks vertically to the right side of the bowl and saucer. Serve all dishes together in the center of the table while keeping extra rice warm on the stove for second helpings. Don't worry about the order in which you eat the dishes: try a little of everything that appeals to you.

Chopsticks: Although it's perfectly acceptable to eat your food with a fork, knife, and spoon, if you truly want to experience Chinese cuisine, use chopsticks. Using them is easier than it looks: first, perch the chopsticks on the first joints of the fourth and middle fingers so that they lie parallel to each other, resting in the crook of the thumb. Secure the chopsticks by laying your thumb on top of them—the lower chopstick should remain more or less stationary while the upper one is maneuvered by the first and second fingers in a pincer movement.

Beverages: Most Chinese drink tea at every meal (see our hints for preparing tea on pages 141 to 142), and often warm rice wine with dinner. However, you may serve the beverage of your choice. Indeed, in more cosmopolitan Chinese cities, whiskey, Western table wines, and just plain water are frequently served. On the other hand, many more traditional Chinese forgo beverages altogether during the meal and then concentrate on finely brewed tea to aid digestion after dinner.

Now that you know something about how to serve your Chinese meals, let's explore what you need in your kitchen in order to prepare the dishes described in Part III.

• *Kitchen Tools*

Chopping Board. You'll need a solid board on which to chop vegetables and cut meats and poultry. A wooden board should be about 11 to 12 inches in diameter and about 2 inches thick. Before you use it for the first time, soak it in water for about an hour, then oil it with olive or vegetable oil to prevent it from splitting.

Cleaver. The cleaver, used to chop vegetables and cut meats and poultry, should be of medium weight and about 3½ by 8 inches in size. A cleaver made from carbon or stainless steel is best for general use.

Steamers. There are two basic types of steamers used in Chinese cooking. Metal steamers act as both water boilers and food containers and sit directly on the burner or heat source. They contain a perforated metal basket that holds the food to be steamed. The traditional bamboo steamer, on the other hand, fits inside the wok that holds the water to be boiled. The wok is placed on a wok rim, which in turn is placed over the heat source. Although both types of steamers do a good job, the bamboo steamer has an advantage as steam is absorbed by the lid rather than condensing and falling on the food making buns soggy or flavors diluted.

Wok. A metal, round-bottomed pan, called a wok, is an essential cooking utensil in Chinese cuisine. Its shape allows heat to spread quickly and evenly, thus allowing food to be cooked with very little fat and in very little time.

Although we think of a wok as a distinctly Asian tool, it works well for all types of cuisine. Woks are available in many different sizes (a 14-inch one is best for all-round use) with both wooden and steel handles (you'll need one with metal handles if you're going to use the wok in the oven). All woks come with a wok stand that provides a secure base for cooking.

Before using a wok for the first time, treat it with oil to avoid rusting: heat the wok over high heat, then brush it lightly with oil. Wipe it clean with a paper towel, then repeat the procedure at least two more times. Then, when you've finished cooking, simply wipe any remaining food from the wok with a paper towel. I prefer a simple heavy-gauge carbon steel wok.

• *Ingredients*

Thanks to the proliferation of specialty markets and increasingly diverse grocery stores, you should have little trouble finding most of the ingredients used in Part III's recipes. If you have trouble, feel free to contact one of the mail-order companies listed in the Resource Guide on pages 215 to 220.

In the meantime, here's a brief description of the most common ingredients in Chinese cooking:

Beans and Bean Products

Beans play a prominent role in Chinese cooking. Virtually any bean is chock-full of protein, complex carbohydrates, fiber, B vitamins, iron, and potassium. At the same time, beans are usually very low in fat and sodium and have the additional benefit of being relatively inexpensive. Beans may be processed into sauces, fermented, or made into a paste.

Bean Curd, Fresh. Fresh bean curd—also known as tofu—is a mixture of finely ground soybeans and water. It has a spongy quality and tends to soak up the flavors of whatever spices and herbs you cook with it. You can find tofu in most grocery stores—usually sitting out in a tray of water—and as part of most salad bars. But be aware that if tofu is left in the open air for too long, it can become a breeding ground for bacteria. To lower the risk of eating contaminated bean curd, heat it for two minutes in boiling water before using it.

Bean Curd, Puffed. The Chinese often deep-fry fresh bean curd to use in dishes. Like fresh bean curd, deep-fried bean curd also absorbs the flavors and juices in a dish while adding protein and texture.

Black Beans, Fermented. Fermented black beans are whole soybeans preserved in salt and ginger. They have a pungent taste, and when cooked with other foods and spices, they lend a rich, earthy flavor to the dish. Black beans are highly nutritious, and especially rich in iron and protein.

Red Bean Paste. Made by mixing sugar with mashed azuki beans (another protein-rich bean), this paste is used most often as a sweet filling for desserts.

Szechuan Chili Paste. Used to spice up dishes, this thick sauce is made by mashing dried red chilis with crushed yellow soybeans fermented with salt, wheat flour, and sugar. This is a highly nutritious flavoring since chili peppers contain lots of vitamin C and soybeans are rich in protein.

Cereals, Grains, Noodles

Now that we in the West have come to realize the importance of complex carbohydrates in the diet, the Chinese way of eating makes much more sense to us. As discussed, rice or noodles serve as the centerpiece of the average Chinese meal, with meats and vegetables in relatively small quantities as accompaniments.

Long-grain Rice. This white grain has been a staple of the Chinese diet since the twelfth century B.C. To cook rice properly, you need the right amount of water, about 12 ounces for each cup of uncooked rice (which makes about 3 cups of cooked rice). First, wash the rice in three or four changes of cold water, then drain and put it into a saucepan. Add the oil and water, cover, and bring to a boil. Stir thoroughly with a wooden spoon, then continue to boil it until most of the water is absorbed. Reduce the heat and allow the rice to simmer for about 12 to 15 minutes. Long-grain rice is neutral in nature and has a sweet flavor; it is often prescribed in Chinese medicine as an energy tonic for the spleen-pancreas and stomach.

White Glutinous Rice. Also called sticky rice, this type of rice, which is more rounded in shape than the long-grain variety, becomes sticky when boiled. The Chinese use it for both savory and sweet dishes, as well as in stuffings for chicken and other game. You can cook white glutinous rice using the same method described for the long-grain variety, but it is preferable to soak the rice for one hour before hand. Sticky rice is warm in nature, but otherwise acts on the body the same way as the long grain variety.

Egg Noodles. Made of wheat flour, egg, and water, these noodles are the most common type used in both Chinese and Western cuisine. Chinese egg noodles, however, tend to be a little more elastic and chewy in texture than the American and Italian types.

Rice Noodles. Rice flour is used to make these tender white noodles used in many Chinese dishes. If you buy dried rice noodles, soak in boiling water until soft or follow the directions on the package.

Dried Products

The Chinese use a variety of dried foodstuffs in their cooking. Mushrooms and dried fruits lend flavor and texture, while cornstarch and agar help to thicken sauces and absorb flavors.

Cornstarch. As its name implies, this white powder is a starch extracted from corn. It is used as a thickener.

Lily Buds. Dried buds of the tiger lily, a flower that grows in abundance in Northern China, these delectable tidbits absorb the tastes of other ingredients while adding a bit of crunch to whatever dish they're in.

Mushrooms. Mushrooms are highly nutritious vegetables, offering about 15 percent of the Recommended Daily Allowance for iron, 35 percent for niacin, and 28 percent for riboflavin. Dried mushrooms—including Chinese black mushrooms, straw mushrooms, and tree ears, to name just a few varieties—are staples of Chinese cuisine. Before you add them to a dish, soak them in warm water for several minutes to reconstitute them.

Herbs and Spices

Considering how flavorful and rich Chinese cooking tastes, you might be surprised at how few spices you'll use in each dish. Indeed, traditional Chinese cooking is quite elegant and simple.

Chili Powder. Chili peppers come in many different colors, shapes, and degrees of hotness. In their fresh form, they're used quite often in Szechuan cooking, which tends to be spicier than cuisines of other parts of China. Whole dried chilis are used or chili powder, made by pulverizing dried chilis, may be added to any number of dishes.

Coriander. Also known as Chinese parsley or cilantro, this is a refreshing and aromatic herb used both as a garnish and a seasoning. It is also available in ground powder form, but in that state has different qualities and flavors. In its dried form, coriander adds a musky, pungent taste to a dish, while fresh coriander has a bright, almost mintlike flavor and consistency. Like its Western cousin, parsley, cilantro contains relatively high amounts of vitamins A and C.

Five-Spice Powder. This seasoning consists of five and sometimes six ground spices including star anise, cassia (Chinese cinnamon), cloves, fennel seeds, and Chinese peppercorns. Sometimes ginger and cardamom are also used. Five-spice powder is often used in marinades for meat and fish.

Garlic. Garlic is an indispensable ingredient in Chinese cuisine and, indeed, in cuisines from around the world. It is rich in vitamins and enzymes invaluable to health and healing. Studies have shown that garlic oil inhibits the coagulation of blood and reduces "bad" cholesterol (low-density lipoproteins, or LDL) while increasing "good" cholesterol (high-density lipoproteins, or HDL).

Ginger. Ginger comes in two forms: ginger powder and fresh ginger root. Although they cannot be substituted for one another, both forms are spicy hot in taste. Fresh ginger root is often used to counter rank odor in a dish, such as fishiness or a heavy garlic smell. From a Western medicine perspective, ginger acts as an anti-inflammatory and helps to boost HDL and lower LDL.

Scallions. Scallions, or spring onions, form one of the three basic condiments in Chinese cooking, along with garlic and ginger. Scallions have long white bulbs topped by green leaves. Different parts of the plant are used in different recipes as you'll see in Part III.

Sesame Seeds. Tiny, flat seeds from the sesame plant, sesame seeds in their whole form add a crunchy texture to dishes. Either white or black, these seeds may also be ground whole into a butter or shelled and milled into a paste called sesame tahini.

Shallots. All onions are a good source of fiber and provide a fair amount of potassium. This member of the onion family is smaller and milder than its cousins the Spanish and Bermuda onions. It is almost a cross between garlic and onion and tends to have a sweet flavor.

Star Anise. Tasting a bit like licorice, this star-shaped, hard spice is frequently used in Chinese cooking to flavor meat and poultry. It is also used to make warming teas.

Vegetables and Fruits

The Chinese use vegetables and fruits extensively in their cuisine. Thanks to the quick and easy method of stir-frying, these fresh foods retain their flavor and texture, as well as their nutritional and medicinal value in Chinese dishes.

Bamboo Shoots. Bamboo shoots are cultivated for consumption in China, but are only occasionally found in their fresh form in the West. However, canned bamboo shoots are available in most grocery stores and add a delicious smooth but crunchy texture to dishes. Fresh shoots must be peeled and parboiled before their use in cooking. Bamboo shoots have a cold energy that neutralizes the effects of the warm or hot energy in meat.

Chinese Broccoli. Also called Chinese kale *(Brassica)*, this leafy vegetable tastes more like asparagus than broccoli. It has a cooling nature and pungent flavor and Chinese medicine practitioners often prescribe it to alleviate summer heat conditions.

Chinese Chives. Chinese chives are darker green in color, more fibrous in texture, and have a stronger flavor than their American cousins. You can find them in Chinese markets. Chives influence the kidneys, liver, and stomach; dry damp conditions; and increase qi circulation.

Chinese Flowering Cabbage and Chinese White Cabbage. These delicate, leafy vegetables look and taste nothing like the cabbage we serve here in the West. Flowering cabbage, which has tiny, edible yellow flowers, has a subtle taste and is chock-full of vitamins and minerals, including calcium. Chinese white cabbage, also called bok choy, is sweet and juicy with a consistency somewhat like that of Swiss chard. Bok choy contains one third of the daily requirement of vitamin C and one half of that of beta-carotene. Just as in the West, the Chinese consider this and all types of cabbage to be good sources of roughage, which helps keep the digestive tract working properly.

Ginkgo Nuts. Once a sacred tree of China, the ginkgo, also called silver apricot, produces fruit with pits that, when peeled, offer tender, mild nuts used extensively in Chinese cooking. Ginkgo nuts are available canned in Chinese groceries.

Hair Seaweed. Rich in nutrients and with a porous texture that allows it to absorb other flavors, hair seaweed is sold in dried form here in the United States. You'll want to reconstitute it in hot water with a few drops of oil before adding it to any dish. Seaweed has a cooling nature and salty flavor that works to detoxify the body, moisten dryness, and build the yin fluids.

Taro. Taro is a root vegetable with a dark-brown skin and a gray or purple flesh. It has a rather glutinous, smooth texture when cooked. Like other root vegetables, taro is considered to have a neutral nature and a sweet and mildly pungent flavor, affecting the stomach and large intestine.

Water Chestnuts. Water chestnuts, which are the bulbs of a sedge plant cultivated in swampy paddy fields or in muddy ponds, provide a crunchy texture to meat and vegetable dishes. In Chinese medicine, water chestnuts have a cold nature and sweet flavor that help to relieve fever and indigestion and affect the lungs and stomach.

Winter Melon. A wax gourd with flesh that turns white when cooked, the winter melon is used often in both Chinese medicine and Chinese cooking. It has a cool nature and sweet flavor that affect the lungs, bladder, and small and large intestine.

Sauces and Oils

One of the added health benefits of classic Chinese cuisine is how little fat you'll need to use to cook most dishes. However, you should be aware—as discussed in Chapter 2—that fat is not considered the "evil" it is here in the West, but simply another energy that should be used in moderation and balance.

Fish Sauce. Made from fish, salt, and water, this golden-brown sauce adds a nice fragrance and taste to a variety of dishes.

Hoisin Sauce. This sauce is made from soybeans, wheat flour, salt, sugar, vinegar, garlic, chili, and sesame oil. You can use it as a dip as well as a marinade or ingredient in savory dishes.

Oyster Sauce. Oyster sauce is made from oyster juice, wheat flour, cornstarch, and white glutinous rice. It tastes less salty and strong than soy sauce.

Peanut and Sesame Oils. Both peanut and toasted sesame oil are used quite often in Chinese cooking. They lend flavor and smoothness to dishes and, in Chinese medicine, are known to lubricate the internal organs.

Soy Sauce. Soy sauce is made from fermented soybeans and wheat or barley, salt, sugar, and yeast. It is perhaps the most basic and common condiment in Chinese (and, indeed, most Asian) cuisine. There are two types of soy sauce: thick soy sauce, which is relatively heavy and sweet in taste, and thin soy sauce, which is thinner and saltier in taste.

• *Cooking Techniques*

Steaming. Steaming involves holding food above boiling water (sometimes combined with spices or rice wine) and allowing the steam to cook the food. Compared with other methods, steaming tends to bring out generally subtler but fresher flavor and textures. There are two major types of steamers used in Chinese cooking. A traditional *bamboo steamer* is placed inside a wok, with the food resting inside it. Boiling water is poured to within 1 inch of the top of the container of food. A *metal steamer* is an "all-in-one" piece of equipment. Made of stainless steel or aluminum, it usually includes a lower container for water and one or two perforated containers that hold the food above it. There are two ways to use steamers. You fill the bottom part with water, place the food and flavorings on a heatproof dish inside the perforated container or steamer basket above the water, then cover the steamer with a tight-fitting lid and set the pot to boiling. You can also put the food directly into the container.

Stir-frying. Stir-frying involves cooking meat, vegetables, herbs, and spices quickly in a small amount of oil and/or other liquid. Because the foods cook rapidly, it's important that you dice your vegetables and prepare your meat before you start to heat the wok.

That way you won't overcook one type of food while you're cutting up another.

— —

Now that you're more familiar with Chinese cooking equipment, ingredients, and techniques, it's time to take a look at how food (and the way you prepare it) can help stave off or alleviate disease. In Part II, we describe thirty-one common conditions and examine them from an East/West perspective.

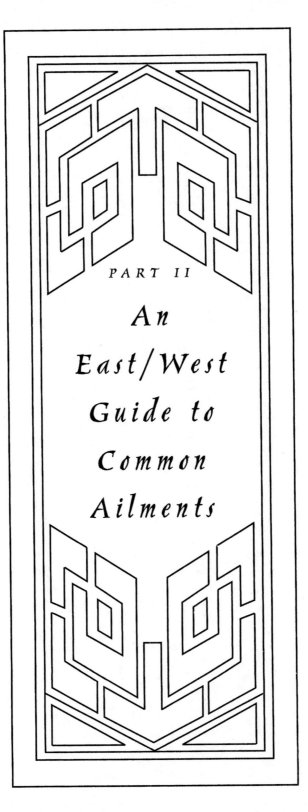

PART II

*An
East/West
Guide to
Common
Ailments*

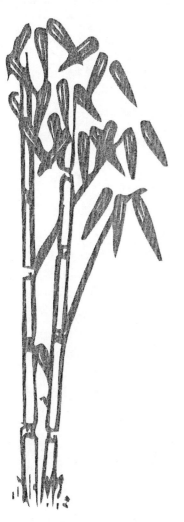

*A*s Part I illustrated, Eastern medicine offers a very different path to health and healing than the one our more familiar Western medicine offers us. In Part II, we look at some of the most common health problems Americans face today and give you a perspective on their causes and treatments from both a Western and an Eastern perspective. Some of these conditions are relatively minor (like bad breath and colds), while others are potentially more serious and debilitating (like arthritis and hepatitis).

Keep in mind that this book is not meant to provide you with all the answers to your medical questions, or to offer you certain "cures" for whatever ails you. That's why it's important for you to visit a qualified health care provider whenever you feel ill. The information in this book is designed to supplement whatever treatment your doctor might recommend as well as offer you a new way of looking at food and how it affects your health. Once you've gained that knowledge, you can apply what you've learned by preparing the recipes in Part III.

• *Anemia*

Are you feeling run-down? Do you lack energy? Are you more prone than usual to develop infections? If so, you may be suffering from anemia, a common and usually easily treatable blood condition. Anemia involves an inability of the blood to carry oxygen to all your body cells. This lack of oxygen results in a variety of symptoms, usually quite mild at first. As the disease progresses, you may notice that you feel more tired than usual and run out of breath more quickly, and that your skin, especially in your nail beds and under your eyelids, is paler than normal. Your heart may beat faster than usual, too.

Both Eastern and Western medicine offer a number of effective treatments for this condition.

From a Western Perspective

Anemia is a general term referring to a shortage of red blood cells or a reduction in their hemoglobin content. Hemoglobin is the pigment in the blood that carries oxygen. Iron deficiency is the most common cause of anemia. It results from a shortage of the mineral iron, which is necessary to produce hemoglobin. This shortage can be caused by a number of conditions, including drastic blood loss (such as after an accident), chronic blood loss (such as with a bleeding ulcer), and certain infections. Women are particularly susceptible to iron-deficiency anemia because of regular loss of blood during menstruation as well as the additional amount of iron required by the fetus during pregnancy. By far, however, most cases of iron-deficiency anemia are caused by a diet lacking in good sources of iron, such as dark green vegetables, egg yolks, meats (especially liver), fish, seafood, and dried peas and beans.

A deficiency of folic acid—a B vitamin also required for hemoglobin production—is another common cause of anemia. Folic acid deficiency is frequently caused or aggravated by malnourishment or alcoholism, as well as by intestinal disorders like inflammatory bowel disease. Less common causes of anemia include diseases that destroy red blood cells (hemolytic anemia), inherited or acquired blood abnormalities (for example, sickle-cell and pernicious anemia), and the failure of the bone marrow to manufacture sufficient numbers of red blood cells (aplastic anemia).

Treatment: Standard medical treatment for anemia depends entirely on its cause. Aplastic anemia, for instance, requires treatment with blood transfusions while pernicious anemia, which involves an inability of the body to absorb vitamin B_{12}, calls for vitamin injections. When it comes to iron-and-folic-acid-deficiency anemias, any underlying problem, such as a bleeding ulcer or an intestinal infection, is diagnosed and addressed first. Depending on how severe the condition is, a doctor might prescribe iron or folic acid supplements. In most cases, a doctor will recommend dietary changes such as those discussed below.

Nutritional Prescriptions: Eating a balanced diet based on the Food Pyramid (see Chapter 2) should provide you with all the vitamins and minerals your blood needs to stay healthy. If you have iron-deficiency anemia, make sure you eat plenty of fresh, raw vegetables. The body absorbs the iron from fresh vegetables more easily than from cooked ones, especially leafy green vegetables, which are especially rich in iron and other essential nutrients. If you are not a vegetarian, you might want to increase your normal intake of egg yolks, liver, and lean red meat—but remember to monitor your cholesterol and fat intake as well. If you're a vegetarian, be sure to eat lots of dried beans and whole grains. Make sure, too, that you eat plenty of foods rich in vitamin C (citrus fruits), as well as niacin-, zinc-, and copper-containing foods (shellfish, nuts, liver, chocolate, raisins, and dried beans), which help the body to absorb iron.

Foods to avoid include coffee, soda, and tannin-containing herbal teas. Caffeine and tannin both tend to reduce iron absorption, as well as to flush excess water from your system, which could lead to a loss of important minerals and vitamins like magnesium and vitamin B_6.

From an Eastern Perspective

In Chinese medicine, anemia is considered a primary symptom of a vacuity of blood, or "weak blood." This blood vacuity is caused by a deficiency in the spleen-pancreas, heart, liver, and/or kidney. Chinese medicine also recognizes that weak blood is the result of iron deficiency, but practitioners believe that this deficiency is caused most often by the inability of the spleen-pancreas to transform qi correctly. Deficiencies of the heart and liver are also common culprits.

Treatment: Acupuncture treatments for anemia concentrate on fortifying the blood and spleen-pancreas. As for herbal remedies, there are several from which to choose, and a practitioner of Chinese medicine would base his or her prescription on your specific constitution and symptoms. Perhaps the most common Chinese herbal remedy for anemia is called *gui pi wan,* or Returned Spleen Tablets. This formula is made of several herbs, including astragalus, ginseng, and tuckahoe. This formula fortifies the spleen-pancreas and the blood, and calms the heart. Once the spleen-pancreas function returns to normal, the body will be able to absorb adequate amounts of iron. *Du huo (Angelica pubescens)* and *hsi hsin (Asarum sieboldii)* are both warm, pungent herbs that help to clear internal heat.

Nutritional Prescription: Foods that supplement the blood and fortify the spleen-pancreas include eggs, beef, liver, red and green pepper, and dates (both red and black). Garlic and ginseng are substances known to overcome stagnant qi and strengthen and energize the blood.

Healing Recipes for Anemics:
Buddha's Delight
Hoisin Beef with Red and Green Peppers
Beef Essence
Bok Choy with Garlic
Steamed Custard with Garlic Chives and Shrimp
Ginseng Chicken Soup
Pork Liver with Garlic Chive Flowers

• *Arthritis and Rheumatism*

Arthritis, or inflammation of the joints, is one of the most common chronic conditions suffered by men and women around the world. Together with other rheumatic conditions that affect muscles and other soft tissues, arthritis represents the leading cause of physical disability in the United States. Symptoms range from mild aches and discomfort to debilitating pain and disfigurement. In both Western and Chinese medicine, arthritis and rheumatism are considered degenerative conditions, which means that symptoms often worsen with time and sometimes spread to other joints in the body.

From a Western Perspective

Arthritis and rheumatism are general terms for more than thirty different conditions, all of which involve the inflammation of one or more joints. Inflammation is the response of the tissues of the body to irritation, injury, or infection. Redness, heat, swelling, and pain are its chief signs.

The two main types of arthritis are osteoarthritis and rheumatoid arthritis. Osteoarthritis, also called degenerative joint disease, is by far the most common of all arthritic diseases. More than half of the adult population over the age of thirty will have some features of this disease, and the percentage increases with age. Osteoarthritis results from a breakdown of tissues, specifically the cartilage between the two bony surfaces that make up a joint. Without the cartilage, bones rub directly against each other. This friction causes the ends of the bones to thicken and form irregular growths called spurs. Spurs can interfere with the joint, causing it to jam or lock.

Doctors are still unsure about what causes the cartilage to break down, but they think a combination of factors is involved. The disease frequently occurs in response to repetitive stress or trauma to a joint over time, but various unknown biochemical and mechanical problems—including defects in the cartilage itself—are clearly implicated as well. Both osteoarthritis and rheumatoid arthritis tend to run in families, which means that genetics also plays a role.

Rheumatoid arthritis, which affects 5 to 8 million Americans, usually strikes people in their thirties and forties and tends to affect women more severely and often than it does men. Like most forms of arthritis, pain and stiffness of the joints are its primary symptoms, and these symptoms tend to be worse in the morning and lessen as the day progresses. However, in many cases, the disease is a systemic one, causing chronic inflammation in the whole body as well as the joints. Symptoms of weakness, loss of appetite and weight, and exhaustion are common. Doctors believe this general malaise represents the body's response to some of the toxic products that result from the sustained inflammation characteristic of the disease. Unlike osteoarthritis, rheumatoid arthritis is an autoimmune disease, which means the immune system actually turns against the body and attacks the joints and possibly major organs such as the heart, lungs, and eyes.

A related disease called gout also causes joint inflammation. Gout results from a buildup of uric acid, a protein present in blood and urine. Normally, the body excretes any excess uric acid but with gout, the acid forms crystals in the joints that rub against the tendons and bones, causing inflammation. Some people with gout also experience other forms of arthritis; others do not. Ninety percent of gout sufferers are men older than forty. Overindulgence in red meat and alcohol may increase the risk of developing gout.

Treatment: As is true for any chronic disease without an identified cause, effective medical treatment of arthritis tends to be difficult. Two general classes of drugs are used in the treatment of arthritis: those designed to relieve pain and inflammation (nonsteroidal anti-inflammatory drugs, or NSAIDs) and those intended to limit or modify the progression of the disease. Both have unpleasant and sometimes dangerous side effects, including intestinal discomfort and bleeding (NSAID); skin rashes, kidney damage, anemia, and nausea (disease-limiting drugs); weight gain, an increase in appetite, high blood pressure, bone loss, and even mental disturbances (steroids).

Nutritional Prescription: Physicians make several recommendations about diet and arthritis. First, you should lose weight if you're too heavy to relieve any stress extra weight puts on your joints. The best way to lose weight is to cut down on saturated fats, increase the amount of vegetables, fruits, and complex carbohydrates in your diet, and, above all, increase the amount of safe exercise you perform each day.

Foods rich in vitamins A, B, C, and E—mainly green leafy vegetables, citrus fruits, and fish—help reduce inflammation, while minerals like calcium, iron, zinc, copper, and manganese are the raw materials the muscles and bones need to stay healthy and repair themselves. Fruits and vegetables also aid uric acid excretion.

Foods to avoid include those of the nightshade family, such as tomatoes, potatoes, eggplant, and peppers. Many people with arthritis are allergic to nightshade foods, which tend to trigger the inflammatory response. Another plant of the nightshade family is tobacco. Not only might tobacco cause an allergic reaction, but nicotine has been shown to reduce blood flow to the muscles and spine, further complicating matters for arthritis sufferers. If you smoke, stop. Although nicotine addiction is one of the toughest to break, the health benefits of doing so are incalculable. Ask your doctor for advice.

In addition, if you suffer from gout, some experts recommend that you limit foods containing purines, substances from which uric acid is formed, including meat, poultry, organ meats, shellfish, mushrooms, and asparagus. Alcohol, caffeine, and chocolate should also be avoided, since they can stimulate the production of uric acid.

From an Eastern Perspective

In traditional Chinese medicine, both rheumatoid arthritis and osteoarthritis are know as *bi* (or blockage) syndromes, in which qi becomes blocked at the joints. In most cases, the qi blockage is caused by a combination of wind/damp. If the joints are very painful and symptoms become worse in the winter, then the blockage is probably caused by wind/damp. When heat is the cause of arthritis, there is swelling and heat in the joints.

Treatment: During the diagnostic procedure, the practitioner of Chinese medicine attempts to determine your particular pattern of internal disharmony. If you suffer from cold arthritis, the doctor will prescribe warming herbs to clear the wind and dampness. A useful herb for treating arthritis is known among Taoists as "food of the immortals." Called *huang jing (Polygonatum cirrhifolium),* this herb helps bolster the health of bones, joints, and muscles, and by so doing, alleviates the symptoms of arthritis as it retards aging.

Individuals with arthritis and rheumatism should try to avoid adverse climatic conditions like wind and damp.

Nutritional Prescription: Most Chinese practitioners would make many of the same dietary recommendations as their Western counterparts, although for some different reasons. From this perspective, it's important to avoid a diet rich in animal fats because these fats promote wind/damp obstructions and thus contribute to pain and inflammation. Foods that drive out wind/damp include basil, cinnamon, fennel, ginger, sage, and black beans. These substances should be added to your diet.

In addition to the recipes in Part III, you might enjoy making a tea with cinnamon twigs and fresh ginger boiled in water for about ten minutes and drink it three times each day.

Healing Recipes for Arthritis:
Poached Fish in Rice Wine Sauce
Silk Squash with Oyster Sauce
Soy Sprouts with Beef

• *Back Pain*

More than 80 percent of Americans will suffer from back pain at one time or another during their lifetimes. This one ailment alone costs us about $30 billion per year in medical expenses, lost wages, and disability claims, and is the cause of 200,000 surgeries every year and countless hours of pain and frustration. Indeed, chronic back pain is one of the most difficult medical conditions to diagnose and to treat today.

From a Western Perspective

There is no one cause of back pain: muscle fatigue and overuse; injury to the muscles, tendons, or ligaments of the back; back spasms; inflammation of the muscles and fascial covering (called myofascial pain); osteoporosis (a decrease in bone density due to the loss of minerals); joint inflammation; misalignment of the vertebrae; herniated or ruptured discs; and pinched nerves are the most commonly identified causes. But it must be noted that in the vast majority of back pain cases, no cause is ever identified.

Treatment: As you might imagine, there is not a lot that modern medicine can do to relieve chronic back pain. Aspirin and non-steroidal anti-inflammatories (NSAIDs) remain the mainstay of treatment, but these merely dull the pain and do nothing to relieve the cause. Exercise and stretching may help, especially under the guidance of a trained physical therapist. Strengthening the stomach muscles, which help provide support to the lower back, is crucial. For those who are overweight, losing weight reduces strain on the muscles of the back that support the spine.

Nutritional Prescription: The general recommendations listed under Arthritis can be applied to back pain as well. Add foods known to help reduce inflammation to your diet, including fresh fruits and vegetables. Make sure you get enough essential vitamins and minerals, especially calcium and magnesium, which work to strengthen the bones and muscles. Protein is also an important building block for muscles and bones, but avoid animal sources since they contain uric acid, a chemical that can build up in the tissues and cause symptoms of arthritis and gout.

From an Eastern Perspective

When it comes to back pain, Chinese medicine holds that the back is governed by the channel of energy called the *bladder meridian,* or the *tai yang* (bladder/small intestine) *channel.* Within the Five Elements system, the bladder is paired with the kidney meridian in the Water element, which is intimately connected with the lower back. Back pain results when the stores of energy held in these meridians and in a reservoir of protective energy called the *governing vessel* that runs along the spine become blocked. Internal heat (inflammation) may also be a culprit.

Treatment: Releasing and strengthening qi along these meridians is the goal of most treatment for back pain. Acupuncture can be especially helpful in this instance. An acupressure exercise that works well to relieve pain involves the following steps: (a) Lie down on your side with your knees bent. Using the flat part of your thumb, stroke up and down along the spinal column from the tailbone to as close to your shoulders as you can reach. Repeat several times. (b) In the same position, stroke downward with your thumb from the top of your spine and then flare outward following the line of the ribs. Repeat this motion several times, then turn over and repeat on the opposite side.

There are several herbal remedies for back pain as well, although it is important to visit a trained practitioner who can evaluate your symptoms and condition before prescribing the right herb. *Du huo (Angelica pubescens)* releases internal heat, *ho shou wu* (Chinese cornbind) reduces inflammation, and *du jung (eucommia)* tonifies kidney energy. If the pain is stabbing, severe, and the affected area feels warm and swollen, the pain is thought to be caused by an obstruction of heat.

Nutritional Prescription: Back pain caused by deficient kidney qi responds to clams and other shellfish, parsley, and sweet rice. Damp heat in the bladder also causes some cases of back pain, and responds to bitter, cooling, and/or alkalizing foods that remove dampness and heat. Winter squash, celery, and mushrooms are recommended. Sweet rice is particularly soothing. Since overeating can intensify heat symptoms, drinking broths and herbal teas rather than consuming heavier foods during the acute phase of a back spasm is suggested.

Healing Recipes for Back Pain:
Beef Essence
Coconut Sweet Rice
Mussels Steamed in Rice Wine

• Bad Breath

There probably isn't a man or woman in the world who hasn't suffered the embarrassment and discomfort of halitosis, more commonly known as bad breath, at one time or another. Its causes are varied and solutions usually quite simple. As you might expect, these solutions often involve an adjustment to your diet.

From a Western Perspective

There are any number of reasons a person develops bad breath. Perhaps the most common is the consumption of animal products (which tend to produce an unpleasant odor) or strong foods like garlic and onions. Poor oral hygiene is another trigger, particularly when it results in tooth decay and gum disease. Bad breath may also occur with upper respiratory tract infections. Some people produce insufficient gastric acid, which can lead to the fermentation of food in the stomach and the exhalation of unpleasant gases.

Treatment: The first step in solving a chronic bad breath problem is to identify and treat any condition that might be the cause, such as an infection or dental problem. If the doctor cannot identify a physical problem, he or she will probably suggest changes to your diet, as well as more scrupulous dental care.

Nutritional Prescription: First, try to identify the foods that cause you the most problems with your breath and try to avoid them as much as possible. Many people find that cow's milk, animal protein, garlic and onions, refined carbohydrates, and coffee are the most common culprits. If you still have a problem, try chewing some natural breath fresheners like parsley, dill, fennel, caraway, or aniseed after a meal.

From an Eastern Perspective

Chinese medicine considers bad breath to be a result of stagnant stomach qi or damp heat in the stomach. If food does not pass through the digestive tract quickly and efficiently, it can ferment or stagnate, thereby producing odorous gases.

Treatment: Solutions for halitosis focus on herbal remedies, such as peppermint tea, radish seeds, and Chinese golden thread, all of which both freshen the breath naturally and also work to unblock stagnant qi. Another herb, called *huang lien* (*mishmi bitter*), also acts to freshen breath, especially when taken as a tea.

Nutritional Prescription: Just as in the West, the Chinese look to the parsley family, which includes cilantro, parsley, and radishes, to help cure bad breath. Citrus fruits, too, especially lemons and limes, have cooling natures and sour flavors that help reduce the effect of internal heat on the stomach and thus ease the digestive process.

Healing Recipes for Bad Breath:
Slivered Radish and Cilantro Salad

• *Bronchitis*

Bronchitis's symptoms include wheezing, fever, and general malaise. Millions of Americans suffer these symptoms every year, especially in the winter when upper respiratory tract infections are most common.

From a Western Perspective

Bronchitis is an infection of the mucous membranes that line the large air passages—the trachea and bronchi—of the lungs. This infection causes the linings to swell up and fill with mucus, making breathing difficult. A harsh cough which often brings up sputum, loss of appetite, fatigue, and occasional vomiting are the debilitating symptoms of this common ailment.

In most cases, bronchitis is the result of the same viruses that cause the common cold. In fact, many people develop bronchitis after a bout with a cold or flu. More rarely, bacterial infections cause bronchitis, in which case antibiotics may be necessary. Most often, however, bronchitis clears up on its own within a few days to a week. It can, however, cause serious breathing problems in small children, so if your child is affected, keep a careful watch on him or her.

Some people develop a condition known as chronic bronchitis, in which the airways become narrowed and partly clogged with mucus that is not moving along as it normally does. Air has trouble entering and leaving the lungs. In almost all cases, chronic bronchitis is caused and exacerbated by cigarette smoking, which irritates the airways, causing them to narrow.

Treatment: Generally speaking, there isn't much that can be done to treat an acute attack of bronchitis, since it's usually caused by a virus, for which there is no cure. Drinking plenty of fluids and adding moisture to the air, however, will help to clear the bronchi and nasal passages. If you have a fever, aspirin or another fever-reducing drug will help to bring it down. You should get plenty of bed rest until the infection passes. If a bacterium is responsible, the doctor will prescribe antibiotics. If you suffer from chronic bronchitis, you *must* stop smoking in order for the condition to clear up. If you don't, you run a much greater risk of developing the life-threatening disease emphysema.

Nutritional Prescription: The best treatment for bronchitis is prevention, which means eating a healthy, balanced diet including plenty of vitamins (especially vitamins C and A, and other antioxidants) and minerals to help keep your immune system in top shape and prevent infections from taking hold. Remember: If you smoke cigarettes, you require at least *three times as much* vitamin C as a nonsmoker. Once you've come down with bronchitis, you might want to try an old home remedy: chicken soup. Chicken contains a natural enzyme called cysteine, which helps to thin mucus. A synthetic version of cysteine, called acetylcysteine, is often prescribed by doctors to treat symptoms of bronchitis, so getting the enzyme in its natural state is sure to help you feel better. If you have a fever, you might want to add some hot pepper or chilis to help you sweat out the infection and to clear out any nasal congestion.

From an Eastern Perspective

Chinese medicine also classifies two different types of bronchitis: acute bronchitis, which is caused by external wind/heat or wind/cold, and chronic bronchitis, which tends to arise because of an internal spleen or lung deficiency.

Treatment: Several different herbs are used to treat bronchitis. For acute bronchitis, your practitioner might recommend *che chien dze* (plantain), a cold, sweet herb that works to clear heat from the lungs and kidneys, or *jie geng* (balloon flower), a neutral, pungent herb that acts as an expectorant and bronchodilator. *Gan tsao* (licorice) is a neutral sweet herb that helps relieve chronic lung and bronchial congestion, as does *hsuan fu hua* (yellow starwort).

Nutritional Prescription: As for the common cold and cough, the Chinese suggest eating less than usual and concentrating on a liquid-based diet when you have bronchitis. Teas made with fresh ginger root and cinnamon may be especially helpful since these herbs help to clear the lungs. Warming pungent foods like mustard greens and bean curd also help to cool and tonify the lungs and clear chest congestion.

Healing Recipes for Bronchitis:
Bean Curd Cubes with Chicken Sauce
Soba Noodles with Mustard Greens

• Candidiasis (Yeast Overgrowth)

Yeast overgrowth, which produces a milky, white rash inside the mouth and sometimes on the genitals, is a common condition, especially among people whose immune systems are working overtime fighting illness or stress. In addition to the rash, candidiasis can trigger food allergies and sensitivities, chronic fatigue and depression, and gastrointestinal problems such as cramps, chronic diarrhea, constipation, and heartburn. Vaginitis (inflammation of the vaginal area accompanied by a white, curdlike discharge), thrush (creamy-white or bluish-white patches on the tongue and throat), and systemic infections of the bloodstream and organs are all potential results of *Candida* overgrowth.

From a Western Perspective

Candidiasis results from an overgrowth of the fungus called *Candida albicans.* This yeastlike substance lives in the bowel, where it helps with digestion, contributes to the bulk of bowel movements, and produces nutrients including vitamin K. At times, however, the balance of microorganisms in the digestive system is disturbed, allowing *Candida* organisms to multiply. Overgrowth is most likely if you are diabetic, produce little gastric acid, or eat a diet based on meat, sugar, and starch and little fiber. Certain medications, including antibiotics, may also trigger a yeast infection.

Treatment: There are several different antifungal drugs, such as nystatin, that can alleviate a yeast-related rash. However, you can only be fully rid of the Candida by addressing the underlying problem. If antibiotics are causing the overgrowth, your doctor should look for another drug or solution to the infection you are fighting. It's important to gain control over diabetes if that seems to be the triggering factor. Bolstering the immune system by eating a healthy, balanced diet can prevent future bouts of candidiasis once you control the initial outbreak.

Nutritional Prescription: Your first step is to try to starve the yeast by cutting out its "favorite foods": added sugar, refined carbohydrates, alcohol, and foods containing large amounts of natural sugar such as milk, fruit, and fruit juice. Garlic, the B vitamins, and fresh, raw, leafy green vegetables will help boost your immune system while acting as antifungal agents. By eating yogurt with active cultures, you can replace the overgrowth of *Candida* with healthier microorganisms: lactobacilli (the microorganisms in yogurt) will colonize the bowel as the yeast dies off.

From an Eastern Perspective

Chinese medicine views candidiasis as a damp illness that causes not only a rash but also fatigue and a weakening of the digestive system as a whole. Anxiety and worry, according to Chinese physiology, greatly contribute to damp excesses such as yeast overgrowth.

Treatment: The herb combination called *she chuang dze tang* (Cnidium Decoction) will help drive out the dampness and energize the kidney and spleen-pancreas. This remedy, which contains *she chuang dze* (Cnidium monnieri) and *gou jidze* (Chinese wolfberry), among other herbs, is especially helpful for vaginal yeast infections. Bitter or pungent herbs such as *tan hsiang* (sandalwood) also help to dry up damp conditions.

Nutritional Prescription: A Chinese practitioner is likely to suggest eating rye, oats, and millet instead of the starchier, more carbohydrate-rich white rice, potatoes, and other starchy vegetables like yams and sweet potatoes. Foods that energize the spleen-pancreas and kidney, drive out damp, and detoxify the body should be eaten regularly. Bitter foods, like the bitter melon dish we suggest here, help drain damp conditions like candidiasis. Foods that help detoxify the body, like bananas, mung beans, cucumbers, and lemon, may also help with this condition.

Healing Recipes for Candidiasis:
Scallops with Long Green Beans
Steamed Stuffed Bitter Melon

Brown Rice with Mung Bean Sprouts and Cabbage Ribbons
Squid with Thin Wheat Noodles in Spicy Sauce

• *Chronic Fatigue*

Extreme fatigue, mild fever, sore throat, painful and swollen
lymph nodes, unexplained muscle weakness and pain—this constel-
lation of symptoms frequently frustrates patients and doctors alike.
In addition to these symptoms, people with a specific disease known
as chronic fatigue syndrome (CFS) also frequently suffer from
headaches, problems with memory and concentration, and sleep
disturbances.

From a Western Perspective

Fatigue can be caused by a variety of conditions, including
anemia, the common cold, flu, and chronic stress. Formerly
known as chronic Epstein-Barr virus (CEBV), chronic fatigue syndrome is an illness believed by scientists to be caused by an as-yet-
unidentified virus.

To date, no laboratory test or x-ray procedure exists to diagnose
CFS, although lab tests may help rule out other problems with similar symptoms like anemia. When evaluating someone with fatigue
that cannot be explained, physicians use the following criteria developed by the Centers for Disease Control to diagnose CFS:

1. Onset of persistent or relapsing fatigue, with at least 50 percent reduction of activity levels for at least six months.

2. Exclusion of other conditions through history, physical exam,
and laboratory tests.

3. Six of the following eleven symptoms: mild fever, sore throat,
painful lymph nodes, muscle weakness, muscle pain, prolonged
fatigue after exertion, headaches, joint pain, neuropsychologic complaints, sleep disturbance, and an acute onset of symptoms.

Treatment: At this time, no known cure exists for CFS. Doctors attempt to alleviate symptoms as they occur, with analgesics and bed rest recommended for pain and exhaustion, and vitamin supplements to help bolster the body's immune system. Magnesium, potassium, and vitamin B complex supplements are especially useful.

Nutritional Prescription: A well-balanced diet like the one outlined in Chapter 2 can prevent, relieve, or lessen the symptoms of chronic fatigue. It is important for you to check with your doctor and a nutritionist to see how your diet might fall short of an optimal one. Maintaining a healthy weight is also important, as carrying too many pounds can deplete your energy as severely as being underweight.

From an Eastern Perspective

The disease called chronic fatigue syndrome is unknown in traditional Chinese medicine. However, it is likely that a Chinese practitioner would consider it to be a disease involving dampness, which, as you may remember from Chapter 1 and the preceding section on candidiasis, is the cause of many chronic conditions.

Treatment: As is true for all damp conditions, chronic fatigue requires exercise in order to oxygenate and "dry out" the body. Overexposure to dampness in the environment may contribute to chronic fatigue, so a Chinese practitioner is likely to suggest you avoid sitting too long outside in the damp, and dressing appropriately if you are regularly exposed to wet cold. Exhaustion in Chinese medicine is often treated with the herbs *ren shen* (ginseng) and *huang chi* (astragalus).

Nutritional Prescription: As is true in the West, protein is thought to help bolster the blood and energize the body, which is why we recommend the following recipes. However, eating too much animal protein could cause you to form mucus, which is considered another symptom of a damp condition like chronic fatigue. You should therefore increase your intake with care and observe any adverse reactions you might have. In fact, the same dietary suggestions given for candidiasis might well be given here: limit the amount of complex carbohydrates and dairy products you consume. Because raw cold foods may contribute to dampness, you should cook your vegetables before you eat them.

Healing Recipes for Chronic Fatigue:
Beef Essence
Five-Spice Pork with Nam Yue

• *Cold Sores*

Unsightly and uncomfortable, cold sores often form on the lips when you are ill with a cold or flu, but sometimes they appear for no apparent reason. They can become a chronic problem in some people, and may be related to stress.

From a Western Perspective

Cold sores are caused by the herpes simplex virus (usually type 1). Once transmitted, this common and highly contagious virus lives permanently in the nerve endings, and thus its symptoms can recur. Any number of things can trigger an outbreak of cold sores, including stress, intense sunlight, another infection like a cold, or simple fatigue. In some cases, an infection may be accompanied by fever. An outbreak of herpes simplex usually lasts about two weeks.

Treatment: There's really not much you or a doctor can do to shorten the course of a herpes outbreak. Try not to touch the cold sore to avoid inadvertently spreading the virus to another spot on your body. Aspirin, acetaminophen, and over-the-counter numbing medicines might help relieve the pain of a sore. Because stress lowers resistance to disease and decreases immune system activity, it leaves you open to a herpes outbreak. You should attempt to manage your stress as best you can with meditation and relaxation strategies if you are prone to stress-related cold sore outbreaks. Getting plenty of rest and regular exercise will also help to keep your body up and running with efficiency and strength.

Nutritional Prescription: Most nutritionists recommend eating foods that contain the amino acid lysine, which helps to slow or alter the growth of the virus. Fish, shellfish, bean sprouts, and fruits and vegetables all contain high levels of lysine. Avoid citrus fruits, however, as they may irritate the cold sore. Other foods you might want to avoid during a herpes outbreak include refined carbohydrates, caffeine, alcohol, and processed foods. These foods may irritate and prolong the infection.

From an Eastern Perspective

Chinese medicine considers damp heat the cause of cold sores. Dampness affects the lungs and stomach, which become congested and produce heat that forms the sores.

Treatment: A practitioner of Chinese medicine might decide to perform acupuncture on points that clear heat and damp from the lungs and stomach. There are several herbal remedies, including *xin yi qingfei yin* (Modified Decoction of Magnolia Flower), which helps to clear the lungs. A topical application to place directly on the sore may be made of *da huang* (rhubarb root) and *huang bai* (philodendron bark).

Nutritional Prescription: Water chestnuts, which are cold and sweet and affect the lungs and stomach, are quite helpful in treating cold sores. Plums can help relieve the sore once it has erupted, as their neutral sweet nature helps treat pain of all kinds.

Healing Recipes for Cold Sores:
Steamed Chicken "Cake"
Chicken Cubes with Lichee and Plum Sauce
Eggplant with Hot Bean Paste
Fish-Filled Wontons

• *Colds and Coughs*

Finding a cure for the common cold and its frequent accompaniment, the cough, is one of medical science's perennial challenges. There's probably not a man or woman alive who hasn't succumbed to the runny nose, itchy eyes, achy muscles, and congestion that accompany the common cold. On average, Americans contract two to three colds per year.

From a Western Perspective

Also known as an upper respiratory infection, the common cold is caused by a virus. Because scientists have yet to find a way to kill viruses, there remains no cure for this temporarily debilitating but otherwise harmless illness. The cold virus—which can live in the air for more than three hours—easily spreads from one person to another through casual contact. You can pick up a virus from an infected person's hands or from contaminated objects—toys, books, telephones, toilet handles, and tables, for example. Once transmitted to the nose or eyes, the virus finds its way into the throat and trachea (windpipe), causing these tissues to become inflamed and filled with mucus. A cold is rarely serious, but in the elderly or chronically ill, it poses an added danger because it can lead to the development of other infections, including pneumonia and bronchitis.

Treatment: Most physicians recommend getting lots of rest, taking aspirin to alleviate fever and aches and pains, and drinking lots of fluid until the virus passes on its own. Prevention, of course, is preferable whenever possible. Getting adequate rest and eating a well-balanced diet that reinforces the immune system are suggested.

Nutritional Prescription: Foods and beverages rich in vitamin C and other antioxidants help to fight infections of all kinds. Garlic has antiviral properties, and thus can be helpful in both preventing the initial infection and clearing it up once it occurs. Drinking lots of clear fluids will help flush out the cold virus more quickly. Avoid milk and milk products, as they produce mucus, which you will probably have an excess of due to the cold. The mineral zinc, if taken at the first sign of infection, may help shorten the duration of a cold.

From an Eastern Perspective

Traditional Chinese medicine considers both colds and flus to be exterior conditions, which means that the disease first affects the body surfaces that are exposed directly to the environment—in this case, the mucous membranes of the nose, throat, and lungs. They can be either a wind/heat or a wind/cold/damp condition.

Treatment: The goal of treatment for colds is to stop the progress of the disease as quickly as possible, which means choosing herbs, spices, and foods that help to push back the wind/damp or wind/heat. Many practitioners suggest sweating out the disease by expanding the sweat glands near the surface of the body.

Herbs to drink as teas include *hsi hsin (Asarum sieboldii),* a warm, pungent herb that helps relieve wind/cold symptoms, especially congestion in the ears and lungs, and *da suan* (garlic), which fights infections of all kinds. One particularly effective formula for most colds and coughs is *geh gen tang* (Pueraria Decoction), made up of several herbs including cinnamon, licorice, and fresh ginger. It makes a delicious tea.

Nutritional Prescription: A practitioner of Chinese medicine would probably suggest eating much less than usual and consuming plenty of liquids. Any number of foods can help relieve colds, depending on the primary symptoms. If chills predominate, you'll want to choose warming herbs and foods, but if you have a fever, you'll want to choose cooling foods. Foods that help bring about sweating, such as cinnamon and hot spices, will also help relieve fever.

Healing Recipes for Colds:
Steamed Carp on Mustard Greens
Cellophane Noodles with Chinese Celery and Cabbage
Steamed Pumpkin with Gingered Honey
Braised Duck with Cinnamon, Garlic, and Bamboo
Fish with Lemon Sauce
Kumquats in Perfumed Syrup
Lo Mein with Mushrooms
Squid with Thin Wheat Noodles in Spicy Sauce
Ginger Tea

• *Constipation*

Contrary to popular belief, constipation does not refer to the *frequency* of bowel movements but rather to their *consistency*. Many people have normal bowel movements only once every other day or two, while some who pass hard, pebbly stools—often larger than normal in diameter—a few times a day are, in fact, constipated. If the stools are particularly hard or large, they may cause tears in the rectum. In cases like these, blood on the stool is not uncommon. In well over 95 percent of all cases, constipation is not a sign of physical illness or abnormality, but rather a problem with diet or other daily habits. Although mild cases of constipation are not serious, chronic constipation can cause a variety of problems, including hemorrhoids, hernias, indigestion, headaches, bad breath, and insomnia.

From a Western Perspective

As discussed, constipation is almost always diet-related, specifically brought on by a poor diet lacking in fluids and roughage. Lack of exercise, which results in insufficient muscle tone in the intestinal or abdominal wall, may be a contributing factor as well.

Treatment: Increasing exercise and improving diet are the two major prescriptions for constipation. In some cases, when all other measures fail, a doctor will prescribe laxatives and/or stool softeners to promote defecation. However, chronic use of laxatives will stimulate the bowel nerves and eventually weaken the muscles. This could worsen and prolong the condition and therefore should be avoided.

Nutritional Prescription: To keep your digestive system working properly, eat a healthy diet as described in Chapter 2. If you've become constipated, try to eat more whole grains, fruits, and vegetables. Bran is the safest, least expensive, and most natural laxative around. You might want to add a little fat to your diet, which will help lubricate your intestines. Garlic might be helpful too, since it contains a chemical called allicin, which stimulates the walls of the intestines. Drink plenty of water—at least six to eight glasses a day. Foods to avoid include milk and cheese, which may cause constipation in some people.

From an Eastern Perspective

Two types of imbalances cause constipation. The most common type is excess constipation, in which constipation results from excessive liver heat or stagnancy. Liver stagnancy inhibits correct qi flow, which in turn slows down the movement of the intestines, and thus the passage of feces. Deficiency constipation, on the other hand, is caused by the lack of yin fluids or blood in the body, which results in dryness and blockage.

Treatment: Practitioners of Chinese medicine choose to concentrate on the diet first, just like their Western counterparts. They also recommend getting plenty of exercise and alleviating stress as much as possible. Again, living a healthy, balanced life in all ways is the fundamental principle here as in all Chinese medicine.

Nutritional Prescription: Foods that lubricate the intestines, including sesame and other oils, as well as cabbage, bean sprouts, and walnuts, will help ease constipation. Foods that help increase yin fluids include black beans, potatoes, and pork.

Healing Recipes for Constipation:
Broccoli with Sesame Dressing
Chicken with Walnuts
Cellophane Noodles with Chinese Celery and Cabbage
Brown Rice with Mung Bean Sprouts and Cabbage Ribbons

• *Diabetes*

Diabetes—a group of diseases related to the body's ability to use food as energy—is one of the most common chronic conditions in the United States. Nearly 14 million Americans suffer from diabetes, and every minute another man, woman, or child is diagnosed with the disorder. It is also one of the most silent diseases known to modern medicine: its symptoms of increased urination, increased thirst, tiredness, and weight loss may be so subtle as to go unnoticed for several months or even years.

If left untreated, diabetes can result in serious health problems, including blindness (it is the leading cause of blindness in people ages twenty-five to seventy-four), kidney disease (every year about 13,000 people are treated for kidney failure related to diabetes), and heart disease and stroke (people with diabetes are two to four times more likely to have heart disease and five times more likely to have a stroke than people without the disorder).

From a Western Perspective

Diabetes is actually a general term for a number of separate but related disorders all involving the body's use of food as energy. Also known as diabetes mellitus, diabetes is caused by either a lack of a certain hormone, called insulin, or the body's inability to use insulin effectively. Insulin is responsible for breaking down the sugar and starches we eat into the body's principle fuel—glucose, or blood sugar. Normally, a little less than half of the carbohydrates and sugar we eat is circulated through the body as glucose. The brain, red blood cells, and muscles use glucose as energy. Some glucose is converted into fat and the rest is stored in the liver for future use.

When the level of glucose rises, the pancreas (a gland that lies behind the stomach) secretes insulin, which helps body cells incorporate and use glucose. In someone with diabetes, however, the pancreas either does not produce insulin or the body does not use the hormone properly. When it cannot utilize glucose due to a lack of insulin, the body starts to burn its own fat and muscle, which results in an accumulation of chemical by-products called ketones.

There are two main types of diabetes. When the pancreas continues to produce insulin but the body cannot use it properly, the condition is known as type II diabetes. It is also known as adult-onset diabetes because the vast majority of type II patients are diagnosed when they are over the age of forty. Type I diabetes occurs when the pancreas produces little or no insulin. Ten percent of people with diabetes suffer from type I diabetes, which is also known as juvenile diabetes because most of those with type I first develop the condition in childhood or adolescence.

Treatment: Treatment of type I involves regular injections of insulin and a strict diet that controls the intake of carbohydrates and sugar. Type II diabetes may be treated with diet and exercise alone or, if the condition remains uncontrolled, with pills or insulin injections as well.

Nutritional Prescription: Diet remains the lynchpin of treatment for diabetes. The one million or so adults and children who have type I diabetes follow a very specific eating plan that works with the insulin they inject during the day to keep their glucose levels as stable and as close to normal as possible.

Diet is just as important when it comes to type II, or adult-onset diabetes, which is by far the more common condition. First, there is ample evidence that being overweight is a major risk factor for the development of the disease. Therefore, by eating a healthy, balanced diet—like the one outlined in Chapter 2—and exercising regularly, you'll help prevent your body from having trouble properly and efficiently metabolizing food. Second, even if you've already developed type II diabetes, you may be able to keep it under control with a healthy eating and exercise plan. You'll want to work carefully with your doctor and, most likely, a nutritionist as well to create a lifestyle that will allow you to control your disease and stay healthy.

From an Eastern Perspective

Diabetes is called sweet urine disease in China because of the high sugar content of the urine of untreated diabetics. Traditional Chinese medicine considers almost all cases of diabetes to be caused by a yin deficiency, often one that involves the spleen-pancreas as well as excess heat in the lungs. As we do in the West, TCM recognizes obesity as a risk factor for diabetes. A high-fat diet is another contributor since it causes liver stagnation, which then causes an imbalance in the spleen-pancreas. Two basic types of diabetes may develop: deficiency-type diabetes, with symptoms of tiredness, pallor, weakness, and poor appetite; and excess-type diabetes, with symptoms of weight gain and constipation along with one or more of the yin deficiency symptoms.

Treatment: Depending on the severity of your disease, a practitioner may well prescribe insulin to help bring your metabolism back into balance. However, dietary measures, an exercise plan, and herbal medicine alone often alleviate the problem. Among the herbs most often prescribed are *huang chi* (astragalus), which works to lower blood sugar; *lung dan tsao* (gentian), which helps to clear heat from the lungs; and *ren shen* (ginseng), which works to regulate blood sugar by fortifying spleen-pancreas and lung energy.

Nutritional Prescription: The goal of nutrition for diabetics is to restore the spleen-pancreas and yin imbalances. For deficiency-type diabetes, a practitioner is likely to recommend that you cook all your vegetables and bolster the spleen-pancreas imbalance by eating plenty of complex carbohydrates. For excess-type diabetes, the practitioner will probably recommend a diet abundant in cleansing foods like raw vegetables and fruits, and foods that are sour and bitter. One general nutritional recommendation your practitioner is likely to make is for you to use oils that contain high levels of omega-3 and other fatty acids, which help protect against heart, eye, and kidney disease related to diabetes as well as bolster insulin's action in the body. Flaxseed oil is a good example of an oil containing omega-3. Foods that are warming and sweet—like pumpkin—benefit the spleen-pancreas.

Healing Recipes for Diabetes:
Chicken Cubes with Lichee and Plum Sauce
Kohlrabi with Swiss Chard Ribbons
Pork Liver with Garlic Chive Flowers
Five-Spice Pork with Nam Yue
Steamed Pumpkin with Gingered Honey

• *Diarrhea*

Loose, watery, and frequent stools are the symptoms of diarrhea, a common condition with myriad causes. Stomach cramps, vomiting, increased thirst, and bloating often accompany diarrhea as well. While a short bout of diarrhea is not often dangerous, chronic diarrhea can result in nutritional deficiencies, especially if loss of appetite occurs along with it. In addition, the change in consistency of the stool causes the body to lose a great amount of water, a loss that can cause dehydration as well as drain the body of essential vitamins and other nutrients.

From a Western Perspective

The most frequent cause of diarrhea is the presence of foreign bacteria in the intestinal tract, often resulting from the improper handling of food. Food allergies, emotional stress, and infections of any type also can result in diarrhea.

Treatment: Unless your doctor diagnoses a serious bacterial infection that can be treated with an antibiotic, he or she will most likely recommend that you simply let the inflammation and irritation run its course. Over-the-counter antidiarrheal medications may ease your situation until the infection clears. If a food allergy is responsible, you and your doctor should attempt to identify the offending substance so that you can avoid consuming it in the future.

Nutritional Prescription: In order to replace the nutrients lost, you should try to eat a diet especially rich in protein, carbohydrates, and vitamins and minerals. Adequate fluid intake is also important, especially for infants and the elderly, who can more easily become dehydrated. Drinks of vegetable juices or hot water with lemon are also recommended. Chamomile tea is both soothing and medicinal. Foods to avoid include milk products, which exacerbate the condition.

From an Eastern Perspective

TCM understands an acute attack of diarrhea to be the body's way of ridding itself of excessive or unwholesome food. Chronic diarrhea, on the other hand, is usually due to weakness in the digestive system, particularly a spleen-pancreas deficiency or excess dampness. There are two types of diarrhea: cold diarrhea, with symptoms that include watery stools, copious urine, and chills; and hot diarrhea, with symptoms that include stools that cause a burning sensation, yellow urine, and a thirst for cold drinks.

Treatment: A TCM practitioner would look first at your diet in order to ascertain what might be causing the internal imbalance or if you are eating too much or too little of a certain food.

Nutritional Prescription: Rice and rice broth, blackberries and blackberry juice, and yams are among the foods known to alleviate diarrhea. Leeks, eggplant, and olives are also helpful because they retard the flow and movement of food through the body. Eggs are especially helpful in treating diarrhea—especially cold diarrhea—because they tend to bind the digestive tract and move qi energy into the upper part of the body. Garlic helps bolster (tonify) the digestive system as well as kill harmful bacteria that may have invaded the intestinal tract. Mushrooms—particularly button mushrooms—are also binding.

Healing Recipes for Diarrhea:
Bok Choy with Garlic
Basic Congee
Ginkgo Nut and Bean Curd Stick Congee
Steamed Custard with Garlic Chives and Shrimp
Eggwhite Crab "Omelet" with Button Mushrooms and Bean
	Sprouts
Ginseng Chicken Soup
Lo Mein with Mushrooms
Oysters Steamed in Egg Custard
Oyster, Mushroom, and Bean Curd Stew
Tea

• *Dizziness*

Dizziness—a feeling of imbalance and vertigo—is a symptom of several different and quite varied conditions. In some cases, dizziness will pass on its own after you eat a bit of food (which raises your blood sugar) or get some rest. When dizziness is chronic or recurring, however, you should seek medical attention.

From a Western Perspective

Chronic dizziness may result from any number of conditions. Some of the more common include untreated hypertension, blood sugar imbalances, including diabetes and hypoglycemia (low blood sugar), an inner ear disturbance called Meniere's disease, and ear infection.

Treatment: Treatment of dizziness depends solely on its cause. If an ear infection is caused by bacteria, your doctor will prescribe an antibiotic. Bed rest and drugs to combat nausea are suggested for Meniere's disease. If your doctor suspects a blood sugar imbalance is responsible for your symptoms, he or she will probably recommend that you undergo a glucose tolerance test at the doctor's office or in a clinic laboratory. After fasting for several hours, you'll drink a sugary liquid, then a lab technician will measure your blood sugar at regular intervals. The results will tell the doctor how well or poorly you use the food you eat as energy.

Nutritional Prescription: Some people with Meniere's disease have been found to be deficient in the B vitamins, so foods rich in B vitamins (whole grains, eggs, lean meats, liver) might be helpful. If you have diabetes, see pages 89 to 91 for dietary recommendations. If you have hypoglycemia, it means that you have abnormally low levels of glucose in your blood, which can be caused by a diet that is too high in refined carbohydrates. In that case, you'll want to avoid heavily sugared foods and reduce foods high in natural sugar. Complex carbohydrates that your body absorbs slowly, like whole grains and vegetables, will help keep a steady level of glucose in your blood. Your doctor will probably recommend that you eat smaller but more frequent meals for the same reason.

From an Eastern Perspective

As in the West, there are several possible causes of dizziness from a TCM perspective, and many of them are related to diet. In most cases, dizziness can be traced to liver heat deficiency.

Treatment: Treatment of dizziness depends on its cause. If liver heat is responsible, several herbs might be helpful. *Lu hui (Aloe vera)* is a bitter herb that acts on the liver and helps to regulate blood pressure. *Du huo (Angelica pubescens)* is another bitter herb that works on the kidneys and bladder to release internal heat.

Nutritional Prescription: Generally speaking, it is important to eat cooling, bitter foods like celery, lettuce, asparagus, and vinegar. These foods will help remove excess heat and restore proper balance to the body.

Healing Recipes for Dizziness:
Cellophane Noodles with Chinese Celery and Cabbage

• Ear Infections

The misery of an ear infection is one that few of us can forget. Pain in the ear, throat, and head; hearing loss; and chills and fever are the main symptoms of an ear infection, although some people experience nausea, diarrhea, and vomiting as well.

From a Western Perspective

Ear infections almost always affect the middle ear—an almost completely enclosed area located just behind the ear drum. The only opening is a small tube (called the Eustachian tube) that leads to the back of the throat—which is why ear infections often spread to the throat and vice versa.

The medical term for inflammation of the middle ear is otitis media. Usually, a bacterial or viral infection is responsible. Sometimes, though, the middle ear fills with fluid because the Eustachian tube is blocked. The doctor must examine the ear drum and the fluid behind it to determine the problem. If the fluid is white and puslike, an infection is probably the culprit. The doctor will take a culture to determine the specific bacteria involved.

Treatment: The two main treatment options include drainage of the middle ear and antibiotic treatment to protect against infection. One way to drain the middle ear is through the Eustachian tube. This is usually accomplished through the use of decongestants. Any infection is treated with antibiotics specific to the bacteria causing the infection.

Nutritional Prescription: Keeping the body well hydrated by drinking plenty of water both counteracts any damage the fever might do and makes the fluid in the middle ear easier to drain. The body also needs vitamins A and C during a fever and to fight infection, so eating plenty of citrus fruits (rich in vitamin C) and fruits and vegetables rich in vitamin A, such as cantaloupe, carrots, tomatoes, and apricots, will help your body recover. Protein also helps the body to repair damaged tissues and fight infection.

From an Eastern Perspective

In most cases, TCM sees ear infections as resulting from a kidney imbalance, usually a kidney yin deficiency. Ear infections also indicate internal cold or heat symptoms.

Treatment: Several Chinese herbal remedies work to fight ear infections. *Hsi hsin (Asarum sieboldii)* is a warm, pungent herb that helps to restore kidney imbalances as well as imbalances in the liver, heart, and lungs. It is especially helpful in alleviating congestion in the Eustachian tubes and upper sinus cavities. If the practitioner believes that internal heat is causing your symptoms, he may suggest using *bo he (Mentha arvensis),* also known as mint, a cool, pungent herb that relieves internal heat conditions in the head and respiratory tract.

Nutritional Prescription: Foods of the mint family such as parsley, peppermint, and spearmint, help relieve internal heat as well as act as pain relievers.

Healing Recipes for Ear Infections:
Basil Coconut Soup with Peppermint Sprigs

• Flatulence

There are few among us who haven't experienced the embarrassing release of gas from the gastrointestinal tract through the colon. Also known as wind, this gas may be accompanied by cramping and bloating. In both the East and the West, flatulence is the most common digestive disturbance.

From a Western Perspective

Flatulence results from a number of different causes, including excess swallowing of air while eating, poor digestion, fermentation caused by bacteria or *Candida albicans* (see page 78) in the stomach, and from certain foods and carbonated drinks. Irritable bowel syndrome, a collection of symptoms caused by irritability and irregularity in the intestines, is another frequent culprit.

Treatment: Treatment of gas depends on its cause. If your doctor finds that you have a yeast infection, he or she will probably suggest some of the measures discussed on pages 78 to 79. Bacterial infections may be treated with antibiotics. You may also find relief from flatulence by taking antacids to reduce the amount of gastric acid your stomach produces. For most cases of chronic flatulence, however, including those triggered by irritable bowel syndrome, you'll probably want to consider changing your diet and eating habits.

Nutritional Prescription: The first thing you'll probably want to do is examine the *way* you eat: Do you gulp down your food? Do you fail to chew slowly and carefully? If so, you could well be taking in excess air that causes your intestines to bloat and gas to develop. If you take some extra time to chew your food carefully and eat slowly, you'll probably experience fewer instances of flatulence. Then, take a look at *what* you eat. Many people find that fatty foods and milk products cause them to have gas. Some people have difficulty digesting very high fiber foods, such as cabbage, apples, cucumbers, and whole grain. The fiber in these foods remains undigested and ferments in the intestine, creating gas. The problem with beans, which are frequent culprits when it comes to flatulence, is that their sugars are difficult to digest. The added air in carbonated beverages makes them problematic for people susceptible to flatulence.

Some flatulence-fighting foods to include in your diet are yogurt and buttermilk, which help to digest high-fiber foods by increasing friendly bacteria in the colon. More efficient digestion will help keep food from fermenting in the stomach and causing gas. Lemon juice and cider vinegar are also recommended for the same reason.

From an Eastern Perspective

Traditional Chinese medicine recognizes stagnation of stomach energy and damp heat as the causes of flatulence in most cases. Another possible cause is liver excess, which affects the spleen-pancreas and stomach functions by invading these digestive organs. The purpose of treatment is to strengthen stomach qi, thus promoting proper digestion.

Treatment: Herbs used to treat flatulence include *rou dou kou* (nutmeg), a warm, pungent herb that acts to reduce intestinal gas and flatulence by stimulating stomach energy. An herb that aids in the digestion of high-fiber foods is *jih shih* (trifoliate orange), a slightly cold and bitter herb that balances spleen-pancreas energy and eliminates damp symptoms.

Nutritional Prescription: A practitioner of Chinese medicine is likely to make some of the same suggestions as his Western counterpart: namely, to eat more slowly and moderately, and to monitor your diet to identify the foods that upset your system. Once you've identified those foods, you can learn to avoid them or work with your practitioner to find combinations of foods and herbs that will aid in the digestive process. If beans cause you trouble, for instance, you may want to cook them with coriander, cumin, and ginger— spices that help to break down high-protein, high-fiber foods and thus prevent the stagnation process from occurring.

Healing Recipes for Flatulence:
Chicken Legs with Pineapple and Mandarin Peel

• *Flu*

Chills, fever, aches and pains, nausea, cough, congestion—these are just a few of the symptoms you experience when you have the influenza virus. Although a bout with the flu is unpleasant, it usually is not serious to otherwise healthy people. The elderly, the chronically ill, and the immune-deficient, however, run higher risks from infection with a flu virus.

From a Western Perspective

Influenza is a contagious disease caused by one of two types of viruses: influenza A and influenza B. Each type encompasses several different strains named for the places in which scientists first identified them, such as the Hong Kong flu and the Russian flu. The tricky thing about a flu virus is that once a strain spreads through a population, it changes in structure and thus can cause a new form of flu. Then, about once a decade, an entirely new strain of flu emerges. Since flu spreads from person to person most easily when temperatures and humidity are low (and we are most likely to be in crowded indoor quarters), most cases occur in the fall and winter months.

Treatment: In most cases, influenza cannot be cured and only the symptoms can be treated, as is true for the common cold. Treatments include bed rest, aspirin to reduce fever and muscle aches, and vaporizers or nasal sprays to relieve congestion.

Nutritional Prescription: In general, you should follow the same nutritional advice given for the common cold and cough on page 85, increasing your intake of fluids and eating a wide variety of whole foods. Even though you might not be hungry, your body needs extra calories in order to recuperate. Foods rich in antioxidants, including fresh fruits, vegetables and garlic, are especially helpful in fighting all kinds of infections, including infection with flu viruses. Vitamin B complex will help your body better metabolize the calories you eat, which is especially important if you lack an appetite. The minerals zinc and iron will help aid the work of the immune system in fighting the infection. Avoid cigarettes, caffeine, and alcohol, which drain your body's nutritional resources.

From an Eastern Perspective

As is true for colds and coughs, flu is considered an *exterior* disease in TCM. In fact, as discussed on page 85, Chinese medicine makes very little differentiation between the two conditions. There are two basic types of flu from this perspective: flu in which fever and other heat signs predominate (wind/heat) and flu in which chills and other cold signs predominate (wind/cold or damp).

Treatment: Treatment depends on which type of flu you have. Generally speaking, wind/heat is treated with herbs and acupuncture designed to relieve heat signs. Among the herbs your practitioner might recommend for wind/heat are *bo he* (mint), which is a cool, pungent herb that works directly on the lungs to expel wind/heat, and *chai hu* (hare's ear), a neutral, bitter herb especially good for colds and flu accompanied by fever and sweating. For flus with primarily wind/cold/damp symptoms, your practitioner might advise taking *hsiang ru (Elsholtzia splendens)*, a warm, pungent herb that helps dispel dampness and wind/cold conditions. *Gan jiang* (dried ginger) is another warm, pungent herb that helps relieve colds and flus with chills. A formula that works for wind/cold flu is *ma huang, fu dze, hsi, hsin tang* (Ephedra, Asarum, Aconitum Decoction). If fever is present but sweating is not, the formula *geh gen tang* (Pueraria Decoction) should help.

Nutritional Prescription: It is quite likely that a practitioner of Chinese medicine, like a Western counterpart, would make the same nutritional recommendations for flu as he or she would for colds and coughs. That is, eat less, drink more, and choose foods that will help counteract your primary symptoms: warming foods if you suffer chills and cooling foods if you suffer fever.

Healing Recipes for the Flu:
Bean Curd Cubes with Chicken Sauce
Steamed Carp on Mustard Greens
Fish with Lemon Sauce
Lo Mein with Mushrooms
Soba Noodles with Mustard Greens

White Fungus in Rich Chicken Broth
Squid with Thin Wheat Noodles in Spicy Sauce
Ginger Tea

• *Hay Fever*

Sneezing, runny nose, watery eyes, itchiness of the eyes and nasal passages, irritability, and exhaustion. If these symptoms sound familiar, you are probably suffering from hay fever. Millions of Americans are plagued with this condition every spring, summer, and/or fall. In advanced cases, they also may experience coughing, wheezing, and respiratory distress.

From a Western Perspective

Hay fever is the term used to describe seasonal allergic reactions to various types of pollen, which are actually the male reproductive cells of flowering plants. Spring attacks are often reactions to tree pollen, summer attacks to grass pollen, and autumn attacks to weed pollen. As is true for all allergies, hay fever represents an overreaction of the immune system to benign substances. What causes this overreaction to occur is still unknown, but research has determined that allergies are genetic, tending to run in families.

Treatment: The best treatment for severe and unrelenting cases of hay fever is avoidance of the triggering substance—even if that means moving to a more urban area that has a lower concentration of airborne pollen. Another technique involves using an air conditioner with a special filter that keeps your home fairly clear of pollen. Several medications can help relieve the symptoms, including antihistamines, which lower the amount of immune system cells that overreact; corticosteroids, which reduce inflammation; and desensitizing shots, which help the body to develop a certain tolerance to pollen.

Nutritional Prescription: Bioflavonoids—substances known as a group as vitamin P—are found in fruits and vegetables, especially those rich in vitamin C. Some bioflavonoids, such as those contained in garlic and onions, work as antiallergic agents, so eating plenty of these vegetables may help relieve your symptoms. Citrus fruits, which contain both vitamin C and bioflavonoids, may act as antihistamines. You might find that hot, spicy foods, such as those made with chili peppers, may help open your nasal passages and relieve chest congestion.

From an Eastern Perspective

The Chinese usually attribute hay fever to an invasion of wind/heat in the lungs, and thus the doctor will attempt to release the lung qi in order to expel the wind heat.

Treatment: TCM might include acupuncture treatments to help relieve the stagnant lung qi. Another remedy a practitioner of Chinese medicine—as well as a Western natural medicine practitioner—may recommend is bee pollen; you would be advised to start taking it about six weeks before and continuing throughout the pollen season. This acts to desensitize the body's immune system the same way that shots given by an allergist would. Herbal remedies that might help restore balance to the immune system include *ma huang* (joint fir, or *Ephedra sinica*), a warm, slightly bitter herb that releases heat in the lungs, as well as *mu dan pi* (tree peony), an herb that also acts to release heat but has a more cooling nature.

Nutritional Prescription: Foods that affect the lungs and airways by clearing heat, such as peppermint, lettuce, and bean curd, serve as soothing remedies.

Healing Recipes for Hay Fever:
Basil Coconut Soup with Peppermint Sprigs
Bean Curd Cubes with Chicken Sauce

• *Headache*

Some of us feel a pounding, others a dull ache, and still others a sharp, splitting pain in the temples or the base of the skull. Headaches stem from any number of causes from the benign to the serious. From both an Eastern and a Western perspective, they remain one of the most stubborn and common health problems.

From a Western Perspective

Headaches are one of the most common medical complaints, sometimes related to a specific underlying condition such as a fever, the common cold or other infection, or a toothache. Most often, however, headaches result from emotional stress or from some unidentified source of tension or physical disturbance. Eye strain due to an uncorrected vision problem may also be the culprit for recurring head pain. Many people get headaches when they are hungry or as part of an allergic reaction to certain foods or substances. Other causes of headaches are high blood pressure and—very rarely—brain tumors or inflammations (encephalitis and meningitis).

Headaches come in all shapes, sizes, and degrees of severity. Migraine headaches, which tend to run in families, are often the most severe and can start as early as childhood. Migraines often occur on only one side of the head and may be accompanied by nausea and vomiting. They can last for hours and rarely respond to aspirin, acetaminophen, or other over-the-counter pain relievers. No one knows what causes migraines to occur.

Treatment: If you have headaches often, you should try to keep a diary to see what you're doing, feeling, and eating just before they occur. If you have a fever with your headache, it's likely that you have a viral or bacterial infection like a cold or ear infection. Your doctor will suggest you bring your fever down with aspirin or another drug, and keep an eye on other symptoms. If a bacterial infection is the cause, your doctor will prescribe an antibiotic. If a head cold or inflammation from allergies is causing your headaches, you might want to try nasal sprays or antihistamines for short-term relief. Your doctor might also test your blood pressure and treat it with exercise, diet, or medication if it is high. Stress is often the cause of headaches, however, and even if your blood pressure is normal, your physician may well suggest you try some relaxation strategies to reduce the amount of tension and stress in your life.

Nutritional Prescription: If your diary shows that your headaches occur after you eat certain foods, it is best that you avoid them as much as possible in the future. If you think your headaches are stress related, you should avoid caffeine and alcohol, which often provoke headaches. Fish oils and ginger may help alleviate headaches, so you should try to increase your intake of these foods.

From an Eastern Perspective

Headaches have many different causes from the TCM perspective. As in the West, these include allergies and food sensitivities, overindulgence in stimulants like caffeine, and colds, flus, and other infections. Most common headaches and migraines are believed to be caused by a stagnation of energy in the liver and gallbladder, which may then invade the stomach.

Treatment: A practitioner of Chinese medicine will ask you to keep track of when your headaches occur and what you think might be triggering them. Acupressure and acupuncture at several points may help relieve headaches. If the practitioner believes that the stomach channel is stagnant, he or she may choose to focus on points on the forehead or along the jaw to bring relief. There are several herbal remedies that might help, depending on the cause. Stagnation of liver qi might call for *lu hui (Aloe vera),* a very cold, very bitter herb that will clear the liver of heat. For nonspecific headaches, perhaps those caused by stress, *du huo (Angelica pubes-*

cens) and *jing jie* (Japanese catnip) are both warm, pungent herbs that affect the liver and kidneys, clearing them of internal heat.

Nutritional Prescription: Liver stagnation and heat, the cause of most common headaches and migraines, are treated with slightly pungent foods and spices, like mint, onions, and sweet rice, among others.

Healing Recipes for Headaches:
Basil Coconut Soup with Peppermint Sprigs
Fishball Soup

• *Hemorrhoids*

Hemorrhoids are enlarged veins inside or just outside the anal canal, which is the opening at the end of the large intestine. As these veins swell, they cause inflammation, itching, and pain.

From a Western Perspective

Several different behaviors and conditions are thought to contribute to the development of hemorrhoids. Chronic constipation may trigger hemorrhoids due to the pressure that straining during bowel movements puts on the veins. Pregnancy may also contribute to the development of hemorrhoids because the enlarged uterus increases pressure on these veins. By far, the most common culprit is a combination of poor diet and poor exercise habits. A diet containing a high proportion of refined foods rather than foods with natural fiber and roughage increases the likelihood of constipation and, therefore, of hemorrhoids. A sedentary lifestyle—one that involves sitting for hours on end, day after day—both increases pressure on the intestinal veins near the anus and contributes to the development of constipation. Being overweight is another common risk factor.

Treatment: Warm baths, over-the-counter remedies, and laxatives may help relieve symptoms, but an increase in exercise and changes in the diet are almost always necessary to resolve the underlying problem. When hemorrhoids are severe, surgery called hemorrhoidectomy may be necessary to remove the dilated portions of the veins. Today, cryosurgery and laser surgery—less invasive but equally effective techniques—are used to remove hemorrhoids, as is rubber band ligation, which involves tying a rubber band around the swollen tissue. A few days later, the hemorrhoid drops off.

Nutritional Prescription: To prevent hemorrhoids from developing, and to reduce the pain of those already existing, it is essential that you eat plenty of whole, unrefined, high-fiber foods which will help keep your bowel movements regular. Cereals, low-fat protein, and fruits and vegetables are highly recommended. Highly spiced food, as well as alcohol, coffee, and other caffeine-rich products, can irritate the bowel and thus should be avoided.

From an Eastern Perspective

In Chinese medicine, a spleen-pancreas qi deficiency usually lies at the heart of hemorrhoid problems. The qi of the spleen-pancreas, often called the "middle qi," helps to hold the internal organs in place: when it is deficient, prolapses such as hemorrhoids can occur. In addition, a combination of heat, damp, and blood stagnation in the anus can be a cause.

Treatment: As well as suggesting many of the same lifestyle suggestions as their Western counterparts, practitioners of Chinese medicine attempt to move the stagnation, cool the heat, and move the blood from the anus, as well as bolster the deficient spleen-pancreas qi. In addition to dietary measures, which we describe next, you may be offered acupuncture to relieve the pain and herbs to bring your body back into balance.

Nutritional Prescription: Foods that correct deficiencies of the spleen-pancreas include most complex carbohydrates and whole grains, which—coincidentally—are the same types of foods Western nutritionists would suggest for this problem. Eggplant is an especially helpful food because it helps to reduce swelling and clears stagnant blood. Low-fat protein sources, like shellfish and beans, help tissues to repair themselves.

Healing Recipes for Hemorrhoids:
Clams and Mussels in Black Bean Sauce
Eggplant with Hot Bean Paste

• *Hepatitis*

Hepatitis, or inflammation of the liver, is a potentially serious condition. Its early symptoms include general fatigue, joint and muscle pain, and loss of appetite. Nausea, vomiting, and diarrhea (or, conversely, constipation) may follow, along with a low-grade fever. As the disease progresses, the liver enlarges and becomes tender. Chills and weight loss also occur, along with the characteristic jaundice, or yellowing of the eyes and skin. Jaundice is caused by a liver malfunction that results in a buildup of bilirubin in the bloodstream. It may also cause the urine to turn brown and stools to become pale.

From a Western Perspective

Hepatitis is an infection of the liver usually caused by one of two hepatitis viruses, hepatitis A and hepatitis B. The most common hepatitis infection is caused by the hepatitis A virus, which is a particularly infectious (contagious) form of the disease. The virus also lives in stools, blood, and saliva; it often is passed on through contaminated food or water. Fortunately, the vast majority of people with hepatitis A infection recover completely, with no permanent liver damage, and run no risk of recurrent infection.

Hepatitis B, on the other hand, is a more serious but slightly less contagious form of the disease. Hepatitis B is transmitted by close mouth-to-mouth contact or from the blood of a person carrying the virus. Infants are sometimes born with hepatitis B virus because their mothers were infected with the virus while pregnant. Among adults, a blood transfusion or injection with a contaminated needle is the most common way for hepatitis B virus to spread. Symptoms of hepatitis B tend to be more severe than those of hepatitis A, and more often lead to permanent liver damage. A complication in about 10 percent of all hepatitis cases is the development of chronic hepatitis, which often involves a lifelong struggle with the disease.

Treatment: There is no cure for viral hepatitis. Once the virus attacks, it's up to your body's own defenses to fight the infection. Plenty of bed rest is essential to help your body stay strong. If you take any medications, please let your doctor know since the liver is responsible for metabolizing many drugs.

Nutritional Prescription: For the most part, eating a balanced diet, such as the one described in Chapter 2, will help you stay as healthy as possible during this time. Drink plenty of water and eat lots of raw vegetables and fruit. It is essential that you avoid drinking alcohol while suffering from hepatitis, since the liver breaks down alcohol during the digestive process and may be further damaged by this effort. Avoid fatty foods because excess fat is stored in the liver.

From an Eastern Perspective

As is the case with many conditions, there is no single category or pattern within Chinese medicine that encompasses all the possible causes or presentations of hepatitis. In many cases, the disease is attributed to the evils of damp heat which invades the liver and gallbladder. Usually, qi stagnation in the liver becomes heat that accumulates in the liver and gallbladder. Heat in the gallbladder results in bile being driven out, producing jaundice. The excess heat then interferes with the functioning of the spleen-pancreas, causing dampness.

Treatment: Several herbs are used by the Chinese to treat hepatitis caused by damp heat in the liver and gallbladder. The choice of which formulas to use is made by a practitioner based on your particular symptoms and body type. Some suggestions he or she might make include *chien tsao* (Indian madder), a cold bitter herb that clears internal heat and acts directly on the liver and heart, and *san chi (Gynura pinnatifida),* a warm, sweet, and bitter herb that tonifies liver energy.

Nutritional Prescription: Bitter foods help improve the general health of the liver as well as drain damp conditions. Among the bitter foods you might want to add to your diet are bitter melon, celery, asparagus, and vinegar. Plums, which are neutral and sweet, are often used to treat liver conditions. Pork helps to strengthen the spleen-pancreas and thus resolve some of the dampness.

Healing Recipes for Hepatitis:
Steamed Stuffed Bitter Melon
Chicken Cubes with Lichee and Plum Sauce
Braised Pork with Black Bean Sauce

• *Herpes Simplex Type 2 (Genital Herpes)*

Blisters that form on the mucous membranes in the genital area are the most characteristic sign of a genital herpes infection. It is a highly contagious disease spread primarily through direct sexual contact. The blister may itch and fill with fluid. Women who suffer from a herpes infection may also develop a vaginal discharge. Both men and women may experience fever and fatigue. As is true for many conditions caused by a virus, genital herpes often recurs.

From a Western Perspective

Genital herpes is caused by herpes simplex virus type 2, which is similar to the virus that causes cold sores on the lips. A diagnosis of genital herpes is based on a visual examination of the characteristic blisters and/or a microscopic examination and culture of the fluid contained in the blisters. Once you are infected, the virus lives inside you forever. However, many people experience only two or three outbreaks—which typically last a week or two—and then find that the virus remains dormant for many years. Stress, colds or other infections, and fevers are some of the more common triggers of a herpes outbreak.

Treatment: Although there is no cure for herpes, there is an antiviral drug called acyclovir that helps to heal the blisters, reduce the pain, and kill large numbers of the herpes virus organisms. In addition, this drug appears to slow the reproduction of the virus in initial outbreaks, thus potentially lessening the number and severity of future outbreaks.

Nutritional Prescription: The same general nutritional suggestions made for cold sores on page 83 would be made here. Eat plenty of foods that contain the amino acid lysine, which has been shown to slow or alter the growth of the virus. Fish, shellfish, bean sprouts, and fruits and vegetables all contain high levels of lysine. If you feel that stress plays a role in your herpes outbreaks, you might want to try either eating more foods that contain vitamin B complex and vitamin E (which are known to help counteract stress in the body) or taking vitamin supplements. Foods to avoid include refined carbohydrates, caffeine, alcohol, and processed foods. These foods may prolong the infection as well as inflict more stress on the body by depleting it of essential substances or filling it with nutritionally empty or even harmful substances.

From an Eastern Perspective

In TCM, herpes is characterized as dampness combined with heat in what is called the "lower burner," the reproductive area of the body. The heat sores that emerge can result from a weakening of the correct qi, which makes the body susceptible to their emergence.

Treatment: Acupuncture at points located on the liver and gallbladder channels would be appropriate in some cases. Herbal remedies include *bai ji (Bletilla striata),* a slightly cold, bitter, and sweet herb, and *shan yao* (Chinese yam), a neutral, sweet herb. Both promote the healing and regeneration of wounded tissues.

Nutritional Prescription: The diet to relieve herpes is a tough one. It involves avoiding all intoxicants (including coffee and tobacco), all sugars, all fruits, all nuts, and all oils except flaxseed oil for a period of about six months, after which these foods can be gradually reintroduced. One of the very best remedies for herpes is tea, taken both internally and applied externally. Indeed, a practitioner of Chinese medicine may suggest that you add six ounces of common black tea leaves to very hot bath water, allow the water to cool, then soak in the water for about an hour.

Healing Recipes for Herpes:
Tea

• Hypertension

Also known as high blood pressure, hypertension may cause either no symptoms or very subtle ones until the problem is quite severe. Among the symptoms you may experience are dizziness, fatigue, and light-headedness. Hypertension causes a myriad of problems in the body, including damage to the heart and blood vessels, which could lead to heart attack or stroke, as well as damage to the kidneys, which must work extra hard to regulate the amount of fluid in the body.

From a Western Perspective

As often as we hear the term *blood pressure,* many of us are unsure of what it really means. In fact, blood pressure is the pressure exerted by the blood as it flows from the heart out to the blood vessels. With each beat, the heart forces 2 to 3 ounces of freshly oxygenated blood into general circulation. Keeping the blood flowing through the 60,000 miles of vessels requires a certain amount of force. This force is called blood pressure. At the head of the blood pressure system is the heart, but the arteries play a large role in determining the amount of pressure in the vessels throughout the body. To raise blood pressure, the arteries narrow; to lower it, they open up. While the force required to keep blood moving through the body originates in the heart and vessels, three other systems—the urinary system (primarily the kidneys), the nervous system, and the endocrine system (which produces hormones)—work together to control blood pressure.

Any number of problems within one or more of these systems may result in high blood pressure. However, in about 95 percent of all cases, no precise cause can be identified. Because the nature of the blood pressure system is so complicated and involves so many components, it is difficult to pinpoint exactly what causes high blood pressure in a given individual. Nevertheless, scientists have identified certain risk factors, including leading a sedentary life, being overweight, and smoking.

Treatment: You can control your high blood pressure by taking one of several different types of medication (each working on a different part of the blood pressure system in a different way) and by making changes in your daily habits. The type and severity of your case of hypertension will guide your doctor in prescribing a course of treatment for you. Depending on your current health habits, you may need to lose weight, exercise more, and better balance your diet.

Nutritional Prescription: Generally speaking, eating a high-carbohydrate, low-fat diet like the one described in Chapter 2 will help you stay at a normal weight and provide your body with all the nutrients it needs. Many people with hypertension are sensitive to salt, and so should reduce the amount of sodium they eat on a daily basis. Foods rich in potassium, like bananas, fish, potatoes, and orange juice, may be beneficial since potassium plays a role in helping the kidneys eliminate sodium from the body. You should also eat lots of celery, garlic, and onion, and fish rich in omega-3 fatty acids (such as salmon and mackerel), all of which help lower blood pressure and keep your heart and arteries healthy. Whenever you use oil in cooking or salad dressing, use olive oil, which helps reduce the level of "bad" cholesterol in the blood vessels.

From an Eastern Perspective

In Chinese medicine, most cases of high blood pressure can be traced to a depletion of kidney energy and/or heat in the liver. Interestingly enough, heat in the liver is fueled by the overconsumption of alcohol and tobacco, and fatty foods like meats and cheeses—the very foods likely to cause cardiovascular problems and obesity, which are the root causes of most cases of hypertension from a Western perspective.

Treatment: As is true in the West, Eastern physicians see hypertension as a disease caused largely by one's lifestyle: the food you eat, the exercise you perform, and the state of relaxation you reach on a daily basis. If you eat too much of the wrong kinds of food, if you don't exercise enough, or if your stress levels are too high, an imbalance like the one that causes a depletion of kidney energy (and thus hypertension) can take place. Therefore, a practitioner of Chinese medicine will not only recommend dietary changes, but also will suggest that you exercise and perform meditation or other forms of relaxation in order to heal your body.

He or she may also recommend one or more of these herbal remedies: *da dzao* (Chinese jujube), a neutral sweet herb that nourishes the blood; *dang sheng (Codonopsis dangshen),* a warm sweet herb that works directly to lower blood pressure as well as nourish the blood; or *yu ju* (Solomon's seal), a neutral sweet herb that acts on the kidneys to lower blood pressure and nourish yin. An herbal formula often used to treat hypertension is *tien ma gou teng yin* (Gastrodia and Uncaria Beverage). Made up of about fourteen different herbs and other ingredients, this remedy acts to dispel the heat and yang excess in the liver.

Nutritional Prescription: Foods that dispel heat signs, like celery and bean curd, and those that help to cleanse the blood, like fish, lemons, and other bitter foods, will help bring your blood pressure system back into balance. As discussed, a practitioner of Chinese medicine is likely to recommend that you eliminate—or at least significantly reduce—your consumption of alcohol, tobacco, and fatty foods.

Healing Recipes for Hypertension:
Cellophane Noodles with Chinese Celery and Cabbage
Ginkgo Nut and Bean Curd Stick Congee
Fish with Lemon Sauce

• *Indigestion*

Indigestion is a very common condition involving painful, difficult, or disturbed digestion. From both a Western and an Eastern perspective, indigestion has many different causes, from simple overeating to food allergies to more serious problems like ulcers or other infections.

From a Western Perspective

Physicians believe that most cases of indigestion occur when either too much or too little gastric acid is produced in the stomach relative to the amount of food you eat. Gastric acid is the substance most responsible for digesting food. If you overeat, your stomach cannot produce enough acid, and so you feel bloated and uncomfortable. If you eat too little, or if you eat foods that stimulate the production of acid, you'll feel queasy and sometimes gassy. Stress, anxiety, or worry can also disrupt your digestion, as can smoking cigarettes and drinking alcohol with meals. In most cases, the symptoms will pass on their own without the need for any treatment apart from the passage of time.

Chronic indigestion, however, may require some investigation by a doctor to root out the cause. Unfortunately, diagnosis is often tricky because the abdomen contains several different organs (the stomach, small and large intestines, liver, spleen, pancreas, kidneys, bladder, gallbladder, appendix, and organs of reproduction). Injury to or infection in any of these organs can cause pain in the abdominal region that resembles indigestion.

Treatment: If the cause of your discomfort is simple indigestion, the treatment usually consists of simply resting quietly until the symptoms have passed. If you feel queasy or gassy, you may want to take an antacid to reduce the excess gastric acid your stomach has produced. If your symptoms are chronic, you may want to discuss the problem with your doctor. It is likely he or she will suggest modifying your diet, by either eating smaller meals or choosing your foods with more care.

Nutritional Prescription: Since each person has a different constitution that is sensitive to different foods and amounts of foods, you may have to reconstruct your diet with a little trial and error to see what's upsetting your digestive system: Is it how much or how fast you eat? Is it what you eat? Until you discover the culprit, you should probably avoid eating too many spicy, fatty, and processed foods and dairy products, since these are the most common problems. Try eating more yogurt, which contains friendly bacteria, as well as papaya, which contains enzymes that can break down protein and other enzymes in the stomach.

From an Eastern Perspective

Chinese medicine views indigestion as signifying a stagnant stomach or spleen qi. Practitioners also recognize the influence of dietary excess, including drinking too much alcohol or coffee, smoking cigarettes, and overindulging in rich, fatty foods.

Treatment: An experienced practitioner might choose acupuncture at several points to treat chronic indigestion, depending on what form the discomfort takes. One herbal treament is *hu jiao* (black pepper), which stimulates stomach qi and thus relieves pain due to stagnation. Both *sha ren* (grains of paradise) and *rou dou kou* (nutmeg) are warm and pungent herbs that act as analgesics (pain relievers) and digestive aids.

Nutritional Prescription: When it comes to nutrition and indigestion, the general watchword in the East, as in the West, is "Everything in moderation." Clearly, if your stomach becomes acutely upset, it's best to eat little or nothing, drink soothing teas, and wait for the spell to pass. However, if you suffer from chronic indigestion, you should choose foods that are soothing to the digestive tract, such as white fish, lemon, and maltose. Eggs and oysters are other good choices. Sweet potatoes are cooling sweet foods, as are radishes and cilantro, which help clear and soothe the digestive tract, as well as tonify the spleen-pancreas.

Healing Recipes for Indigestion:
Five-Spice Roast Duck
Fish-Filled Wontons

Fish with Lemon Sauce
Poached Fish in Rice Wine Sauce
Kohlrabi with Swiss Chard Ribbons
Kumquats in Perfumed Syrup
Oysters Steamed in Egg Custard
Slivered Radish and Cilantro Salad
Sweet Potato Soup

• *Insomnia*

Nothing is more annoying, or ultimately more draining to one's health, than the inability to sleep. The human body, mind, and spirit require sleep in order to regenerate, repair, and reenergize. Lack of sleep is linked to mood disorders, immune system dysfunction, and a host of other physical and emotional ailments.

From a Western Perspective

Generally speaking, Western practitioners view insomnia as resulting from either an emotional disorder such as anxiety, stress, or depression, or a medical problem such as asthma, heart disorders, migraines, or diabetes. Other causes include lack of exercise and the use of drugs and/or alcohol.

Treatment: Although insomnia can be a sign of more serious neurological or physical problems, most cases stem from poor sleeping, eating, and exercise habits. Most doctors first recommend that you examine those issues, then, if all else fails, offer you a mild sedative. Sleeping pills are addictive, however, and you should avoid them if at all possible.

Nutritional Prescription: Foods containing tryptophan, such as tuna, milk, dates, and bananas, eaten just before bedtime, may well help you fall asleep, and stay asleep. There are several herbal remedies as well, such as chamomile, basil, lemon, and valerian. It is very important that you avoid alcohol and caffeine, as both of these substances create hormonal and glucose disturbances that could keep you awake. Simply eating a balanced diet, exercising regularly, and feeling well should solve most problems of insomnia.

From an Eastern Perspective

Traditional Chinese medicine considers insomnia to be a mental disorder, much as depression and schizophrenia are here in the West. Insomnia is considered to be connected to a deficiency of the heart, which houses the *shen,* or spirit.

Treatment: Practitioners of Chinese medicine are likely to suggest ways for you to try to calm your mind and soothe your spirit as the best way to prepare your body for sleep. Meditation and yoga are two very good ways to bring your body and mind into harmony, especially if you learn these methods from an experienced practitioner. There are also several herbal remedies for you to try.

Nutritional Prescription: In some cases, practitioners may suggest you perform a short fast in order to cleanse your system and thereby relieve your mind from the upsets triggered by excesses of any kind. Once you begin to eat again, you should try to focus on foods that help soothe nervousness, such as dates, lily buds, and oysters, as well as those that nurture yin, which is the quiet, peaceful energy in the body and spirit. Yin-nourishing foods include oysters, eggs, and bean curd.

Healing Recipes for Insomnia:
Buddha's Delight with Dried Bean Curd Sticks
Vegetarian Hot and Sour Soup
Oyster, Mushroom, and Bean Curd Stew
Oysters Steamed in Egg Custard

• *Menopausal Symptoms*

The menopause—the end of a woman's fertility—also marks a dramatic decline in her natural secretion of the essential hormone, estrogen. In addition to the cessation of menstruation, menopause may cause serious side effects, such as an increased risk of heart disease and osteoporosis, as well as a host of more minor but nonetheless troublesome symptoms, such as hot flashes, skin changes, mood changes, and headaches.

From a Western Perspective

Here in the West, menopause is a passage marked by a host of sociological, political, and psychological imperatives. Until very recently, this society tended to look at late life not as a treasured and respected life stage, but as a time of physical and mental deterioration and gradual social inconsequence. We've often considered the loss of fertility to also involve the loss of sexuality, vitality, and health.

Fortunately, times are changing, and for two reasons. First, advances in medical science mean that more women and men are living longer and healthier lives. Second, baby boomers—those people born between 1945 and 1960—make up the largest segment of the population, and they're passing through menopause in greater numbers every year. Thus, if only as a self-protective measure, society at large is taking a more benevolent and optimistic look at late life and finding ways to make those years as healthy and vital as possible.

Treatment: That said, the decline of estrogen production does indeed have serious health and aging consequences for a woman's body. As stated, estrogen is important not just in terms of fertility, but also in maintaining the health of the cardiovascular system, the strength of the bones, and the integrity of the skin, hair, and nails. In fact, many scientists now look upon menopause, and the aging process in general, as a medical condition that can be treated by replacing the hormones that are lost as we age, in this case estrogen.

Estrogen replacement therapy, or ERT, has become the standard treatment for menopause. Women take pills made of synthetic or natural forms of estrogen and, usually, progesterone, the other female hormone that diminishes as we age. Women who take ERT appear to suffer much lower rates of heart disease, osteoporosis, and menopausal symptoms like hot flashes and vaginal dryness than women who do not. However, ERT does not come without risks, including higher risks for breast cancer and endometrial cancer.

If a woman decides not to take ERT, there are other ways to help prevent the complications and side effects of menopause. Regular, strenuous exercise is probably the best prescription for women entering or passing through menopause. Exercise helps maintain a healthy body weight, strengthens the bones, fortifies the cardiovascular system, and lessens stress, anxiety, and depression.

Nutritional Prescription: A well-balanced diet, one that allows you to maintain a healthy weight and obtain essential nutrients, is key to passing through menopause easily and in good health. In addition, you will probably need to supplement your dietary intake of calcium, magnesium, and vitamin D—all substances required for proper bone metabolism. Vitamins E and A help keep mucous membranes moist, which helps alleviate the vaginal dryness that often occurs.

From an Eastern Perspective

The Chinese view menopause as a natural change that should, but does not always, go smoothly. When hot flashes and other side effects occur, a practitioner of Chinese medicine sees this as a sign of a yin deficiency.

Treatment: Several herbs nourish yin, including *dang gui (Angelica sinensis),* which is used to treat all kinds of problems related to menstruation and the female cycle—and is thus known as the "Great Tonic for All Female Deficiencies." *Dzang hung hua* (Tibetan saffron), a slightly bitter, pungent herb, helps bolster the yin, heart, and liver, while the herbal formula *jia wei shiao yao tang* (Enhanced Eliminate and Relax Decoction) helps alleviate such common menopausal symptoms as nervous tension, headaches, dizziness, insomnia, and depression. This formula contains *dang gui (Angelica sinensis), bai shao* (white peony), and *chai hu* (hare's ear), among other herbs.

Nutritional Prescription: A diet rich in foods that bolster the yin energy will help you pass through menopause with less discomfort. Interestingly enough, the same kinds of foods and nutrients suggested by the Western approach apply here as well. Foods rich in vitamin E, such as wheat germ and wheat germ oil, help keep mucous membranes moist, while soy products, including bean curd, soy milk, and miso, help build yin. Foods that encourage fluid movement and thus moisten dryness, such as mussels and clams, are also recommended. A practitioner of Chinese medicine will also recommend that you increase your intake of calcium, magnesium, and other vitamins and minerals that help protect the health of your bones.

Healing Recipes for Menopausal Symptoms:
Ginkgo Nut and Bean Curd Stick Congee
Mussels Steamed in Rice Wine

• *Menstrual Problems*

Headaches, backaches, constipation, breast tenderness, mood swings, abdominal pain extending to the hips, lower back, and thighs—these are the most common symptoms of premenstrual syndrome, and millions of women all over the world suffer with PMS and other menstrual problems to some degree. The blame for this discomfort can be placed on the female cycle itself, which involves the ebb and flow of several different hormones that cause significant changes in every part of the body and mind. Some women experience symptoms at the time of ovulation, when an ovary releases an egg and sends it through the fallopian tubes into the uterus. Most women, however, experience problems the week before and then during menstruation, when the uterus prepares to expel an unfertilized egg.

From a Western Perspective

Dysmenorrhea is the medical term for painful menstruation. The cramping of the uterus as it expels its lining is usually the source of this disturbance. Some research suggests that an overproduction of prostaglandins, hormonelike fatty acids that help stimulate uterine contractions, might be the root cause of the discomfort in many women.

Treatment: Traditionally, doctors have suggested analgesics such as Tylenol, Motrin, Advil, and a host of other over-the-counter pain relievers to ease this monthly discomfort. To reduce water retention and bloating, physicians can prescribe a diuretic, but because you can become dependent on diuretics, you should use them only as a last resort. Some women find that taking oral contraceptives, which release a steady flow of hormones to mimic their natural cycle, may help relieve symptoms. Oral contraceptives, however, have their own set of side effects and risks—including increased risk of breast cancer—and thus may not be the best approach for all women. Without question, regular exercise, which keeps the muscles of the body strong and lithe while boosting mood-enhancing endorphins, makes many women feel better before, during, and after their periods.

Nutritional Prescription: By avoiding salt in the last few days before your period, you can reduce bloating and fluid retention. If you also avoid caffeine, you may feel less irritable and tense and have less of a problem with breast soreness. Vitamin B_6 is helpful for overall symptoms, vitamin E is useful for breast tenderness, and fiber and the B complex vitamins help alleviate constipation. Eating complex carbohydrates helps boost levels of serotonin, a brain chemical known to relieve depression and anxiety.

From an Eastern Perspective

Generally speaking, Chinese medicine considers menstrual problems to be a result of an imbalance of liver, spleen, and kidney energies. As is true for menopausal symptoms, PMS may also involve a yin deficiency.

Treatment: Acupuncture, especially with moxibustion, is often very effective for PMS and its symptoms. In addition to a good diet and regular exercise, a practitioner may recommend meditation and yoga to relieve stress.

Several herbs are also helpful, including *dang gui (Angelica sinensis)* and *yi mu tsao* (leonurus, or Siberian motherwort), which are both reliable all-around remedies for female reproductive system disorders. *Gan tsao* (licorice) helps detoxify the body while bringing the hormonal system back into balance. As Daniel Reid points out in his excellent resource, *A Handbook of Chinese Healing Herbs,* Chinese practitioners have known about licorice's remarkable healing properties for more than 1,400 years: Chinese physician Sun Ssu-mo wrote that "the detoxifying power of licorice when it meets poisons in the human body can be compared to the melting power of a pan of boiling hot water when poured onto snow on the ground."

Nutritional Prescription: A practitioner of Chinese medicine is likely to prescribe foods to help relieve constipation and bloating as well as to build yin.

Healing Recipes for Menstrual Problems:
Chicken with Walnuts
Chicken Cubes with Lichee and Plum Sauce
Ginkgo Nut and Bean Curd Stick Congee
Mussels Steamed in Rice Wine

• *Nausea*

At some point, almost everyone experiences the queasiness and impulse to vomit that are the hallmarks of nausea. Some of us feel it while we're pregnant; others while traveling in a boat, plane, or even an automobile; still others after eating or drinking too much. In both Eastern and Western medicine, nausea is not a disease, but a symptom of an underlying problem.

From a Western Perspective

Although we think of nausea as a condition that arises from the stomach and intestines, the vomiting reflex is actually controlled at a site in the brain stem known as the vomiting center. Any number of conditions and situations can activate the vomiting reflex, including motion sickness, food poisoning, viral or bacterial illness, many different kinds of drugs, certain foods, emotional distress, and unpleasant odors, sights, and sounds. Nausea is also common in the first three months of pregnancy.

Treatment: Generally speaking, if the nausea is short-lived and related to an identifiable cause, it is probably no cause for concern. In that case, lying down until the symptoms pass or taking an antacid if nausea is accompanied by gas or cramping may be sufficient. If other symptoms are present, such as high fever, diarrhea, and/or profuse sweating, or if the nausea is chronic and persistent, a more serious underlying cause may be responsible; you should see a doctor for a thorough examination.

Nutritional Prescription: Until the nausea passes, it is best to eat simple, low-fat foods in relatively small quantities. Drink plenty of clear liquids, including distilled or bottled water, and herb teas, especially chamomile and ginger, which soothe the stomach. Avoid coffee, citrus juices, and alcohol, which can irritate the gastrointestinal tract.

From an Eastern Perspective

According to TCM, the most common causes of nausea are food stagnation and stomach qi that flows upward, counter to its normal downward direction. Nausea may involve disharmony of either or both the spleen-pancreas and stomach, and there may also be liver involvement.

Treatment: For nausea due to overeating, a particularly helpful herbal formula is *bai he wan* (Preserver Harmony Pill). For food stagnation caused by a spleen-pancreas disharmony, a formula such as *jian pi wan* (Strengthen the Spleen Pill) might be more effective.

Nutritional Prescription: As is true in the West, Chinese practitioners are likely to recommend that you keep your meals small, simple, and light. Congee, a gruel made of rice, helps to tonify qi energy and calm the digestive system, making it one of the best and most nutritious foods for treating nausea. Ginger also helps to harmonize the stomach and reduce nausea, although you should take it in moderate amounts if you also have a fever, since ginger is a warming herb.

Healing Recipes for Nausea:
Basic Congee
Ginseng Chicken Soup
Kumquats in Perfumed Syrup

• *Pain, Chronic*

The poet Emily Dickinson once wrote:

> Pain has an element of blank;
> It cannot recollect
> When it began, or if there were
> A day when it was not.

Her words describe the seemingly endless and debilitating condition of chronic pain, pain that occurs continuously, sometimes for no apparent reason, sapping your strength and resolve, clouding your optimism and spirit, undermining your health. Chronic pain can result from any number of underlying conditions, from arthritis to infection to a previous trauma (e.g., accidents, surgery) to cancer. But some people suffer chronic pain in the absence of any past injury or evidence of body damage.

Indeed, pain is a very individual matter, involving complex physical and psychological variables, and the pathway of pain is a complex one. When you burn your finger on the stove, for instance, the sensation of pain travels along a series of nerve fibers from your finger to the brain. And there are many ways that the pain message may be altered or even canceled along the route. From both an Eastern and a Western perspective, the goal of therapy is to prevent the pain message from arriving in the brain or dulling the brain's perception of pain should the message arrive.

From a Western Perspective

Here in the West, we usually think of pain as something acute, a response to an injury that resolves itself once the injury has healed, and for most people, that remains true. But for a number of different reasons, pain can become chronic. With a long-lasting and variable condition like arthritis or cancer, for instance, you can literally become "stuck" within the pain, caught in a cycle of frustration, fear, and exhaustion.

Treatment: The doctor's first objective is to establish the cause of the pain. The four most common culprits are a disease or injury, tense muscles from stress or from protecting an injured body part, muscle deconditioning that occurs during long periods of bed rest, and emotional disturbances like fear and depression.

Depending on the cause and the severity of the pain, the doctor might prescribe painkillers, also known as analgesics. Analgesics are either narcotic (such as Percodan, Demerol, and codeine) and act like morphine—by inhibiting pain impulses in certain centers of the brain. Others are nonnarcotic, including aspirin, ibuprofen, and other nonsteroidal anti-inflammatory drugs as well as acetaminophen. Most of these medications inhibit your body's production of inflammatory compounds, called prostaglandins, and are especially useful for bone pain, some types of arthritis, and headaches. All pain medication, however, has risks and side effects. Narcotics may be addictive and also impair physical and mental function. Nonnarcotics may cause skin rashes, digestive upset, and blood thinning.

Most doctors, even in the West, now look for other solutions to chronic pain problems. The use of heat, cold, and massage is sometimes helpful. These three applications work by stimulating the skin and other tissues surrounding the painful area, which, in turn, increases blood flow.

Unless you've suffered a severe injury or illness, your doctor is likely to suggest a safe exercise program. Exercise is known to stimulate the production of endorphins, natural chemicals produced in the spinal cord and brain that operate in the same manner as narcotic analgesics.

Nutritional Prescription: It is very important that you eat a well-balanced diet rich in vitamins and minerals so that your body stays

strong and has all the raw ingredients it requires to repair and reju-
venate. Fruits and vegetables contain anti-inflammatory substances,
so eating more of your favorite produce may help. You should stay
away from caffeine, as it may interfere with the natural painkilling
actions of endorphins, and tobacco, which reduces blood flow to the
muscles.

From an Eastern Perspective

In most cases, chronic pain is caused by a blockage or other disruption in the flow of qi through the body. A practitioner of
Chinese medicine first attempts to locate the source of the pain and
then to understand the underlying imbalance causing it. As you may
remember, traditional Chinese medicine considers the chronic pain
caused by arthritis, for instance, to result from blockage of qi at the
joints, usually caused by excess wind and dampness.

Treatment: The approach to treating chronic pain in Chinese medicine depends entirely on the underlying imbalance. Generally speaking, however, acupuncture will probably help a great deal, as it is
known both to block messages about pain from reaching the brain
and to release endorphins. The practitioner would also offer one of
several herbal remedies, again depending on the underlying cause.

Nutritional Prescription: When it comes to diagnosing and treating chronic pain, a practitioner of Chinese medicine would spend a
great deal of time assessing whether your diet helps to keep your
body in balance or is creating an underlying disturbance that is the
reason for your pain. He or she would then create an eating plan that
would address any imbalances. One food particularly helpful for
cases of chronic pain caused by inflammation is squash, which is a
warm sweet food.

Healing Recipes for Pain:
Silk Squash with Oyster Sauce

• *Psoriasis*

This skin condition, which produces patches of red, scaly skin, affects about 1 percent of the U.S. population. It tends to be a chronic and troublesome condition that first appears in early adulthood. It frequently occurs after an injury to the skin or a generalized infection, and once it has appeared it can be precipitated or aggravated by emotional stress, drug reactions, or infections such as strep throat.

From a Western Perspective

Doctors in the West are still mystified as to the cause of psoriasis. There seems to be a genetic predisposition to the disorder in many patients, and it is somehow related to a defect in the production of the epidermal (top) layer of the skin. Instead of taking the usual twenty-six to twenty-eight days for the epidermis to form, the process takes only three to four days. This causes an abnormal outer layer of skin that we see as round or oval patches of skin covered with silvery or red scales.

Treatment: Psoriasis remains a difficult and problematic condition to treat and to date there is no cure. You can find temporary relief in the form of corticosteroid creams or ointments, coal tar preparations, and ultraviolet light—in fact, as long as you put sunscreen on the rest of your body, a day of sunbathing can do wonders for your psoriasis. Your doctor can also arrange for you to undergo medically supervised ultraviolet light therapy. Other treatments may include acid gels or creams for the removal of scales and anti-inflammatory medicine for any discomfort.

Nutritional Prescription: Most nutritionists would suggest that you cut down on the amount of meat and fat you eat, as these contain substances that interfere with the way your body uses essential fatty acids to maintain healthy skin. Bolster the amount of natural oils and moisture your skin and other tissues have available: Eat plenty of oily fish like mackerel and salmon, and massage primrose oil and linseed oil into the affected areas of the skin. Several nutrients play important roles in skin health, including vitamin A, the B complex, vitamin C, vitamin D, and zinc. Some researchers have found vitamin E—taken internally or externally—to be very effective in healing psoriasis.

From an Eastern Perspective

In traditional Chinese medicine, the skin has a close relationship with the lungs and the blood. The lungs are both the source and distributor of qi, which circulates beneath the skin. The blood nourishes and moistens the skin, and disorders of the blood often manifest themselves as skin problems like psoriasis. It is thought that wind becomes trapped between the interior and exterior layers of skin.

Treatment: The Chinese find it just as frustrating to treat psoriasis as we do here in the West. Acupuncture treatments designed to release the trapped wind may help, as may treatments that help relieve stress that could trigger an attack. One of the most effective herbal remedies—from both a Western and an Eastern perspective—is *lu hui (Aloe vera)*. Aloe vera is helpful in healing all types of skin problems. It is available in many forms, including a condensed juice, a tea, and an ointment. Another herb that will alleviate psoriasis is *bai ji (Bletilla striata)*, which helps promote healing and regeneration of wounded tissues.

Nutritional Prescription: Cool, lubricating foods, like sesame and sesame oil, help provide the skin with the moisture it needs and counterbalances the excess heat often involved in the problem.

Healing Recipes for Psoriasis:
Broccoli with Sesame Dressing

• *Sinus Infections*

Throbbing pain of the face and temples, stuffiness, fever—these are the most common symptoms of a sinus infection, a condition that recurs periodically for millions of Americans.

From a Western Perspective

The word *sinus* is the medical term for a cavity. There are sinuses in many parts of the body, but the ones people are most familiar with are those in the bones around the face. The sinuses (of which there are four primary pairs around the nose and eyes) are connected through small openings into the nasal cavity. Any infection or inflammation in the nasal cavity, such as the common cold or an allergic reaction, can cause tissue to swell in and around the sinus openings, leading to blockage. Blocked passages often lead to infection, since the sinuses are unable to flush away bacteria or other toxins.

Treatment: The first item on the agenda is tracking down the cause of the inflammation and infection. If the cause is viral, you'll simply have to wait out the disease process by drinking plenty of fluids and resting (see other suggestions under Colds and Coughs on page 85). If the doctor has reason to believe a bacterial infection is the culprit, he or she might prescribe an antibiotic. Decongestants may help both relieve the pressure and pain and allow drainage of the offending microbe from your sinuses.

If you suffer from chronic sinus infections, your doctor may suggest you keep track of when they occur to see if an allergic reaction might be a trigger. In rare cases, if the problem is severe and chronic, your doctor might recommend that a surgeon enlarge the sinus openings or create a new drainage hole.

Nutritional Prescription: As is true for any infection involving the nasal passages, you should steer clear of dairy products, since they promote the creation of mucus that further blocks the sinuses.

Spicy, hot foods help relieve stuffiness, as does the old standby, chicken soup. Adequate intake of vitamins A and C helps to fight infections of all kinds. Potassium, calcium, and zinc are thought to aid the work of the cilia, the tiny hairs in the nasal passages that help expel mucus.

From an Eastern Perspective

From a traditional Chinese medical perspective, qi deficiencies of the lung usually cause sinus infections. As is true for colds and coughs, sinus infections are considered exterior conditions and can either be a wind/heat or a wind/damp condition.

Treatment: Treatment focuses on pushing back the wind/damp or wind/heat and bolstering the lung's qi deficiency. If your sinus problems are chronic, your practitioner may suggest ongoing acupuncture to resolve the underlying imbalance. To treat acute symptoms, he or she may suggest some herbal remedies, including *mu tong* (akebia) to help relieve sinus congestion, *du huo (Angelica pubescens)* to push back wind/damp or wind/heat, and *bo he* (mint) to tonify lung qi and relieve wind/heat symptoms in the head and respiratory tract.

Nutritional Prescription: The Eastern nutritional prescription closely resembles the one you might receive from your Western doctor—at least for treatment of the acute symptoms. Concentrate on eating (or drinking) hot spicy foods both to help relieve congestion and to stimulate perspiration and thus reduce fever. Foods rich in vitamin C, garlic, and other antioxidants also help fight infections. For chronic conditions, your practitioner will help you create a healthy, well-balanced eating plan designed to restore and maintain your own unique internal balance.

Healing Recipes for Sinus Infection:
Five-Spice Roast Duck
Five-Spice Pork with Nam Yue
Steamed Pumpkin with Gingered Honey

• *Urinary Tract Infections*

No one who has ever had a urinary tract infection (UTI) will ever forget its symptoms: pain and burning with urination, increased urge to urinate but decreased flow, and, occasionally, fever. Far more common in women than men, UTIs are often chronic conditions requiring frequent treatment.

From a Western Perspective

Urinary tract infections occur when bacteria infect any part of the urinary tract, including the kidneys (which produce urine), bladder (which holds urine), ureters (which transport urine from the kidneys to the bladder), and urethra (which carries urine out of the body from the bladder). In most cases, the infection is centered in the bladder, a condition known as *cystitis*. A urinary tract infection can be serious, and always warrants medical attention. With medication, most UTIs clear up within a week.

Treatment: Treatment for a UTI usually involves taking a course of antibiotics for ten days to two weeks. Chronic urinary tract infections sometimes result from poor toilet habits that bring the urethra into contact with bacteria from feces. Your doctor may suggest that you wash after every bowel movement, as well as after sexual intercourse, since this is another time when bacteria may enter the urethra.

Nutritional Prescription: Drinking plenty of water is the first and most important nutritional remedy a doctor is likely to suggest. Water will help flush out the bacteria more quickly. Cranberry juice, which contains a special enzyme that kills some bacteria known to invade the urinary tract, is also a good choice.

From an Eastern Perspective

TCM holds that qi is necessary to promote smooth and proper flow of fluids within the body, including the production and voiding of urine; most urinary tract infections occur because qi has been disrupted. This disruption may involve damp heat in several organs, including the bladder, kidney, small intestine, spleen-pancreas, and lungs.

Treatment: Treatment includes dietary modifications as well as herbal remedies. One of the best herbal formulas is *ba jeng san* (Eight Orthodox Powder), which is especially useful for UTI caused by internal heat and internal damp conditions. *Di fu dze* (Belvedere cypress) is an herb that acts as a diuretic, or urine producer, which helps to flush out the bacteria from your system.

Nutritional Prescription: Foods that promote urination (like sweet rice) and bitter, cooling foods (like peppers) which help clear out damp heat, might be right for you while you're suffering from a UTI. Lamb is known to strengthen kidney deficiencies and so may help reduce urinary problems.

Healing Recipes for Urinary Tract Infection:
Hoisin Beef with Red and Green Peppers
Spicy Lamb with Wide Rice Noodles
Coconut Sweet Rice
Sweet Potato Soup

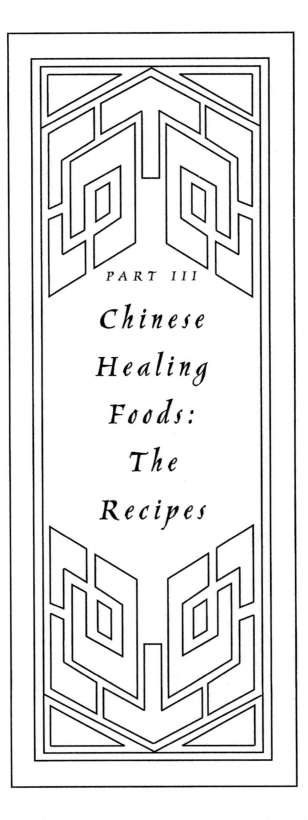

PART III

Chinese

Healing

Foods:

The

Recipes

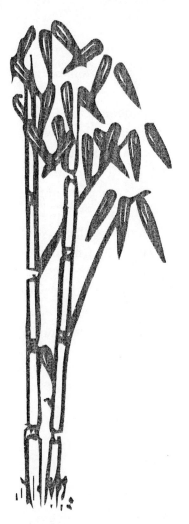

*T*HE FOLLOWING RECIPES ARE designed to be both delicious and healthful. Most are very low in fat, all use a variety of fresh ingredients, and you're sure to find them easy to prepare. Furthermore, each dish is designed to treat a certain condition or conditions according to the principles of Chinese medicine.

Please be aware, however, that these are very general medicinal suggestions. According to Chinese philosophy, you have a unique constitution that requires a very specific balance of energy and nutrients in order to work properly. If you're serious about maintaining your health using Chinese precepts, it's essential that you visit a qualified practitioner of Chinese medicine. Only after examining you with care will he or she be able to prescribe a diet that will maintain your internal balance or correct any disharmonies that may have arisen.

In the meantime, you have nothing to lose and much to gain by trying these recipes—whether you choose to prepare them when you're feeling ill or if you just want to enjoy good, healthful meals. If you find it difficult to locate a specific ingredient, try one of the mail-order companies listed in the Resource Guide at the end of the book or use another ingredient in the same family. In addition, feel free to reduce the amount of oil or other fats in these dishes if you like, especially if you have a nonstick wok or saucepan. Remember, though, that these are, by and large, traditional Asian recipes, and Asians have relatively low rates of heart disease and obesity. If you eat a balanced diet rich in complex carbohydrates, leafy green vegetables, and lean protein, you shouldn't concern yourself too much about a tablespoon or two of vegetable oil in your food.

⊡ *Beverages*

— *Green Tea* —

Tea is the universal drink all over Asia: Asians drink it at most meals as well as to treat specific medical ailments. In recent years, Western scientists have been examining the potential health benefits of green tea, the type most commonly used in China. There could be a substance in the tea that helps prevent heart disease, hypertension, and other chronic conditions that are so much less common in Asia than in the United States.

Good for: Diarrhea, herpes simplex

Healing Properties: Green, red, or black tea leaves have an astringent quality that makes them good for drying up sores like those caused by the herpes virus. In severe cases, practitioners of Chinese medicine make a poultice of tea leaves that have been soaked in hot water and apply it directly to the sore. In both the East and the West, tea is used for cases of diarrhea and indigestion caused by inflammation.

NOTE: For medicinal purposes, tea is usually strongly brewed by simmering the leaves for 30 minutes or more.

1. Warm a porcelain pot (in China, porcelain is always heated with hot water while water for the tea is boiling in a kettle).
2. Discard the hot water in the teapot, add 1 teaspoon of tea leaves per cup, and pour boiling water over the tea leaves. Cover the teapot immediately and let the tea steep for about 5 minutes (see Note).
3. True tea enthusiasts remove the leaves from the water by straining the tea into a clean, warm porcelain pot, but you can sim-

ply pour it from its original brewing pot if you prefer. Most Asians drink tea plain, but you might like to add milk, sugar, or lemon.

— *Ginger Tea* —

This simple tea, made with fresh ginger root, is excellent for colds and coughs. It relieves the feeling of stuffiness in the head and chest that is a cause of so much discomfort.

Good for: Colds and coughs, indigestion, flu

Healing Properties: Ginger is a warm, pungent food that induces perspiration (which helps relieve fever and congestion) and disperses cold. It affects the stomach and spleen-pancreas as well as the lungs, so drinking this tea may also soothe an upset stomach.

PREPARATION: 5 minutes   COOKING TIME: 25 minutes
YIELD: 1 cup

---

1 ounce fresh ginger root, about 10 slices the size of a quarter
2 cups water

1. Peel the ginger and then slice thinly.
2. In a small saucepan, combine the ginger slices with 2 cups cold water. Bring to a boil, reduce the heat, and simmer, uncovered, until the tea reduces by half and tastes strongly of ginger, about 20 to 25 minutes.

🔲 *Soups*

— *Basil Coconut Soup with Peppermint Sprigs* —

This is a delicious soup that you can serve as a filling main course for six people or as a starter course for eight to ten people. Because coconut milk is rich in saturated fat, you should eat this dish only on special occasions, especially if you tend to eat red meat, butter, or other fatty foods often. If you can't find rice vermicelli in your market, regular semolina vermicelli is a good substitute.

Good for: Earache, edema, hay fever, indigestion

Healing Properties: Each ingredient in this delicious soup has its own healing qualities. Basil is a warm, pungent spice that promotes blood circulation and digestion, and is thus ideally suited to help soothe an upset stomach. Coconut milk is a warm, neutral food that helps foster urination and digestion (which makes it helpful in relieving any swelling in the body, including the edema often related to diabetes). Peppermint is a cool, pungent food that affects the lungs and airways (thereby easing the congestion of hay fever) and helps to relieve pain.

PREPARATION: 25 minutes   STANDING TIME: 10 minutes
COOKING TIME: 25 minutes   SERVES: 6 (as a main course)

---

1 pound medium shrimp
4 ounces rice vermicelli (mei fun)
4 cups vegetable or chicken stock
8 basil leaves
10 to 12 peppermint leaves
2 cups unsweetened coconut milk
1 teaspoon salt
½ teaspoon red pepper flakes, or to taste
6 peppermint sprigs

1. Peel and devein the shrimp (reserving shells), placing them in a bowl of ice water until needed.

2. In a small bowl, soak the vermicelli in warm water until soft, about 10 minutes. Drain and reserve.

3. In a saucepan, bring the stock to a boil, add the shrimp shells, and simmer 10 to 15 minutes. Drain and discard the shells.

4. Chop the basil and peppermint leaves into shreds.

5. Return the broth to the heat, add the basil and peppermint leaves, coconut milk, salt, and pepper flakes. Bring to a simmer and cook 5 minutes.

6. Add the shrimp and vermicelli and cook, stirring, until the shrimp just turns pink, about 5 minutes.

7. Spoon the soup into bowls, garnish with peppermint sprigs, and serve.

— *Beef Essence* —

Making this broth is worth all the time it takes as the resulting essence is very strengthening and quite delicious. It's a perfect dish for anyone who's ill, especially someone with little appetite. The slow cooking extracts all the flavor of the meat, but the soup remains clear.

Good for: Anemia, chronic fatigue

Healing Properties: Beef is a warming, sweet food that is used as a tonic for the spleen, stomach, and blood. Eating a concentrated beef soup like this one can bolster the iron in your blood, thereby alleviating anemia and giving you a boost of energy.

PREPARATION: 10 minutes   COOKING TIME: 4 hours
YIELD: 1 quart

---

1 pound lean beef, cut into thin strips
5 slices fresh ginger
¼ cup rice wine
5 ½ cups water
Salt to taste

1. Place the beef and ginger in a pot with a tight-fitting lid. Add the wine and water and bring to a simmer. Do not let it boil.

2. Cook over low heat for 2 hours, adding water if necessary. Cover and continue cooking another 2 hours over low heat or until the broth is flavorful.

3. Strain and discard the beef. Serve the soup flavored with salt to taste.

— *Fishball Soup* —

If you're not feeling well, this is a good way to get your protein. This soup can be made more filling by adding some cooked noodles to it. For a stronger mint flavor—and more medicine for your headache—you might like to add a few more spearmint leaves, roughly torn, to the stock while it is simmering.

Good for: Headache

Healing Properties: Surprisingly enough, spearmint is an excellent remedy for headache, either in a recipe like this one or brewed as a tea. The fish, of course, provides lots of healthful protein and essential fatty acids.

PREPARATION: 20 minutes   COOKING TIME: 15 minutes   SERVES: 6

½ pound flounder fillet
2 water chestnuts
1 scallion, whole
½ teaspoon minced ginger
½ teaspoon salt
½ teaspoon pepper, plus more as needed
4 cups low-sodium vegetable broth
1 teaspoon thin soy sauce
½ cup spearmint sprigs, loosely packed

1. In a food processor, combine the flounder, water chestnuts, and scallion. Pulse to grind well. Add the ginger, salt, and ½ teaspoon pepper, and continue processing until the mixture is well blended and smooth. Wet your hands and form the fish mixture into balls about 1 inch in diameter. Place on a wet plate and set aside.

2. In a saucepan bring the broth to a simmer. Add the fishballs and continue to simmer until they are firm to the touch, about 3 to 5 minutes. Season with soy sauce and pepper.

3. Spoon into bowls and sprinkle spearmint leaves over each bowl. Serve hot.

— Ginseng Chicken Soup —

This is a tasty way of drinking ginseng. If you make a large pot, you can refrigerate or even freeze it to warm up later. If you omit the chicken, you'll have a delightful ginseng tea!

Good for: Anemia, diarrhea, nausea

Healing Properties: Ginseng is one of the most strengthening and energizing food substances in Chinese medicine. For this reason, practitioners often prescribe it for anemia and the fatigue that goes along with it. It is also excellent for soothing an upset stomach, especially in this chicken soup recipe.

> PREPARATION: 5 minutes   COOKING TIME: 4 hours
> YIELD: About 4 quarts

1 whole chicken, about 2 pounds
1 ounce ginseng
2 slices ginger
10 dried red dates

1. Place the chicken in a large stockpot or saucepan, cover with cold water, and bring to a boil. Reduce to a simmer, add the ginseng and ginger, and simmer for 2 hours.
2. If the broth reduces too much and the chicken is exposed, add more water.
3. Add the red dates and continue cooking the broth another hour.
4. Strain the soup and degrease. You can either skin, bone, and slice the chicken so it can be returned to the soup with pieces of ginseng and red dates, or you can serve the soup as a clear broth.

— *Vegetarian Hot and Sour Soup* —

This meatless and healthy version of the ever-popular hot and sour soup will convert even the keenest meat lover.

Good for: Insomnia

Healing Properties: Strangely enough, it's the lily buds in this recipe, tiny plant pods found in Asian markets or through a mail-order distributor, that help you sleep by easing nervousness. If you really have trouble sleeping, you can boil a handful of lily buds in water for half an hour, sweeten with a little sugar to taste, and drink the water at bedtime. The other ingredients in this soup, including the two kinds of mushrooms and the bean curd, provide vitamins, minerals, and protein.

> PREPARATION: 15 minutes   STANDING TIME: 15 minutes
> COOKING TIME: 15 minutes   SERVES: 6

1 tablespoon dried lily buds
1 tablespoon dried tree ears
4 dried mushrooms
¼ cup bamboo shoots, slivered
6 water chestnuts, slivered
4 cups low-sodium vegetable broth
4 tablespoons rice vinegar
2 teaspoons thin soy sauce
1 teaspoon cayenne pepper (or to taste)
½ pound bean curd (tofu), cubed
2 tablespoons cornstarch mixed with ¼ cup cold water
Salt and pepper to taste
2 egg whites, or 1 whole egg

1. In three separate bowls, soak the lily buds, tree ears, and dried

mushrooms in warm water until soft, about 15 minutes. Drain the lily buds and tree ears. Discard the water. Remove the mushrooms from the liquid, reserving the liquid. Stem the mushrooms and cut them into slivers.

2. In a saucepan, combine the lily buds, tree ears, mushrooms, mushroom liquid, bamboo shoots, and water chestnuts with the broth. Bring to a simmer. Add the rice vinegar, soy sauce, and cayenne pepper.

3. Return the soup to a boil and add the bean curd and the corn-starch mixture. Stir gently to mix well, and cook 1 minute or until the soup thickens. Add the salt and pepper. Turn off the heat and imme-diately stir in the egg whites or whole egg with a fork. Serve hot.

— *Spinach and Bean Curd Soup* —

This simple soup can accompany a dinner or lunch. For a heartier soup, add a few pieces of fish or shrimp.

Good for: Anemia, constipation

Healing Properties: Spinach is a cool, sweet food that helps to lubricate dry tissues, making it an excellent remedy for constipation. It is also used as a blood tonic. Western medicine recognizes spinach as the source of a vast quantity of minerals and vitamins, including calci-um and vitamin A.

PREPARATION: 10 minutes   COOKING TIME: 5 minutes   SERVES: 4

---

1 pound soft bean curd (tofu)
3 cups low-sodium chicken stock
2 tablespoons thin soy sauce
½ teaspoon pepper
1 cup spinach leaves, finely shredded
1 teaspoon sesame oil

1. Drain and cut the bean curd into cubes.

2. In a saucepan, bring the stock to a boil, add the soy sauce, pepper, and bean curd. Return to a boil and simmer 1 minute. Add the spinach shreds and cook until the spinach is just wilted and bright green.

3. Remove from the heat and drizzle in the sesame oil. Serve.

— *Sweet Potato Soup* —

Although this soup tastes rich, it is soothing to the stomach and is especially good if you've overeaten the night before. If you want to cut down on the fat, you can replace some or all of the cream with nonfat evaporated milk.

Good for: Indigestion, urinary problems

Healing Properties: Sweet potatoes are cooling, sweet foods that strengthen the spleen-pancreas.

PREPARATION: 10 minutes   COOKING TIME: 1 hour   SERVES: 8

1½ pounds sweet potatoes
3 cups chicken stock
1 head garlic, peeled
1 tablespoon vegetable oil
1½ tablespoons curry powder
2 teaspoons minced ginger
1 cup cream
Salt and pepper to taste

1. Preheat the oven to 350 degrees F. Rinse the potatoes and roast them in the oven for 40 minutes or until tender. Bring the stock to a boil and blanch the garlic for 5 minutes; remove the garlic from the stock with a slotted spoon.

2. Scoop the potato pulp out of the skins. In a food processor or food mill, puree the potato and garlic cloves. Combine them with the stock.

3. Heat the oil in a small saucepan and sauté the curry powder until aromatic, about 2 minutes. Be careful not to let the curry burn. Add the curry and ginger to the soup. Simmer for about 15 minutes. The soup may be prepared to this point and held until you're ready to serve it.

4. To serve, return the soup to the heat, add 1 cup of cream or nonfat evaporated milk, and simmer until the soup is hot. Season with salt and pepper to taste. Serve.

— Cold Tomato and Ginger Soup —

This is an Asian version of the Mediterranean soup known as gazpacho. Its spicy flavors make it a perfert summer lunch or dinner appetizer. It is best made a day ahead and served well chilled. If you like, you can serve it hot in the fall or winter.

Good for: Colds and coughs, constipation

Healing Properties: The ginger helps to relieve congestion and disperse cold, while the cold and sweet tomatoes produce fluids and promote digestion. Rich in vitamin C and antioxidants, this soup can also be a hearty tonic in winter if you serve it hot.

PREPARATION: 30 minutes   COOKING TIME: 15 minutes
SERVES: 8 to 10

---

4 pounds ripe tomatoes
1 tablespoon diced red onion
2 tablespoons grated ginger
1 to 2 cups ice water
Salt and pepper to taste

1. Bring a pot of water to a boil and blanch the tomatoes briefly. Drain and refresh the tomatoes in a bowl of ice water. Peel the tomatoes, cut them in half, and remove all the seeds. Chop coarsely. You should have about 6 cups.

2. In a food processor, puree the tomato pulp, onion, and ginger. Add ice water to achieve the desired consistency. Season with salt and pepper to taste, chill for an hour or overnight, and serve.

3. If you decide to serve it warm, heat the soup gently in a pan over low heat.

— *White Fungus (Snow Fungus) in Rich Chicken Broth* —

This exotic fungus is often cooked with rock sugar and served as a last course at formal dinners. It can also be made with chicken for soup, but if the chicken broth is really rich, this recipe is truly delicious. I recommend making your own broth for this dish.

Good for: Colds and coughs, constipation

Healing Properties: In the East as well as in the West, chicken soup remains one of the best-loved and most effective cold remedies. White fungus helps to lubricate the lungs and is considered an important yin tonic.

PREPARATION: 15 minutes   COOKING TIME: 20 minutes
SERVES: 6 to 8

---

1 package (4 ounces) white fungus (snow fungus)
4 cups rich chicken broth
1 tablespoon dry sherry
Salt and pepper to taste

1. Soak the white fungus in warm water until soft, about 15 minutes. Drain and remove the tough ends.

2. Heat the broth in a deep saucepan, add the sherry and fungus, and bring to a boil. Reduce the heat to very low and simmer for 20 minutes, or until the fungus softens slightly. Add salt and pepper to taste before serving.

— *Winter Melon Soup* —

This everyday version of a soup usually served at formal banquets is both easy to make and good for you. You can buy just a slice of melon to use in this dish.

Good for: Urinary infections

Healing Properties: Because winter melon detoxifies the body and helps promote urination, it is especially helpful in clearing up urinary tract infections quickly.

PREPARATION: 15 minutes   STANDING TIME: 15 minutes
COOKING TIME: 20 minutes   SERVES: 6

1 slice winter melon, about 1 pound
6 dried black mushrooms
1 ounce bean thread noodles
4 cups vegetable stock
2 pieces dried tangerine peel
2 tablespoons thin soy sauce
1 teaspoon black pepper
6 water chestnuts, sliced
¼ cup bamboo shoots, slivered
1 cup ginkgo nuts
2 eggs, beaten
Salt and pepper to taste
Orange zest (optional)

1. Peel the winter melon and cut it into 1-inch chunks. In a bowl of warm water, soak the mushrooms until soft, about 15 minutes. Drain, reserving the water, and remove the stems. Cut the mushrooms into slivers. In another bowl of warm water, soak the noodles until soft. Drain and cut into 5-inch lengths, if desired.

2. In a deep saucepan, combine the stock, tangerine peel, soy sauce, and pepper. Bring to a boil and simmer, covered, 15 minutes. Add the melon, mushrooms, water chestnuts, bamboo shoots, and ginkgo nuts. Cook until the melon is translucent, about 10 minutes. Add the bean thread noodles, and cook another minute.

3. Remove from the heat and immediately stir in the beaten eggs with a fork. Season to taste with salt and pepper. Serve garnished with orange zest for extra flavor.

⊡ *Vegetables*

— *Bean Curd Cubes with Chicken Sauce* —

This dish can be either spicy or mild, depending on your taste.
Omit the chili paste altogether or add extra if you like a little zip!

Good for: Bronchitis, flu, hay fever

Healing Properties: The cooling yin quality of bean curd (tofu) benefits the lungs and thus helps to alleviate bronchitis and flus that
occur with fever. It also helps clear wind/heat from the lungs, which
may help relieve hay fever. If you decide to make the dish spicy, the
chili paste may act to relieve any congestion that accompanies your
infection.

PREPARATION: 15 minutes   COOKING TIME: 15 minutes
SERVES: 2 to 4

¼ pound ground chicken
1 teaspoon soy sauce
1 teaspoon sesame oil
1 tablespoon fermented black beans
1 garlic clove, minced
1 tablespoon peanut oil
4 firm bean curd (tofu) squares, about ½ pound
½ cup vegetable stock
2 teaspoons cornstarch mixed with 1 tablespoon water
½ teaspoon chili paste (optional), or more to taste
1 scallion, minced

1. In a small bowl, combine the chicken with the soy sauce and
sesame oil. Rinse the black beans and mash lightly with the garlic.

Add 1 teaspoon of the peanut oil to the black bean mixture. Cut the bean curd into cubes.

2. Heat the wok, add the remaining peanut oil, and stir-fry the black bean mixture for 30 seconds; add the chicken mixture and continue to stir-fry, making sure to break up the chicken.

3. Add the stock, cornstarch mixture, and chili paste (if you like). Bring to a boil and cook until the sauce thickens, about 5 minutes. Add the bean curd to the sauce, mix well, and cook until the bean curd is warm. Sprinkle with scallions and serve.

— *Steamed Stuffed Bitter Melon* —

Most Chinese love bitter melon, but for many Westerners it is an acquired taste. In this recipe, the sweet shrimp and pork filling balances the melon's bitter flavor. Perhaps you'll find that the savory filling helps make this unusual vegetable one of your favorites.

Good for: Candidiasis, hepatitis

Healing Properties: The bitter melon in this recipe is good for hepatitis because, like all bitter foods, it can improve the condition of the liver. Bitter foods also drain various damp-associated conditions such as candida overgrowth.

PREPARATION: 20 minutes   COOKING TIME: 20 to 25 minutes
SERVES: 4 to 6

---

2 bitter melons, about 1 pound
1 teaspoon baking soda

STUFFING
½ pound ground pork
½ pound medium shrimp, peeled and deveined

1 cup mung bean sprouts, chopped
1 scallion, minced
1 tablespoon sesame oil
2 teaspoons thin soy sauce
1 tablespoon cornstarch
½ teaspoon salt
1 teaspoon ground pepper
3 tablespoons oyster sauce (optional)

1. Cut the bitter melons in half lengthwise. Remove the woody pulp and seeds with a spoon.

2. Bring a pot of water to a boil, add the baking soda, and blanch the melon halves until they turn bright green and begin to get soft, about 5 minutes. (The blanching will help soften the bitter flavor.) Drain and plunge the melons into cold water.

3. In a food processor, combine the pork, shrimp, mung bean sprouts, scallion, sesame oil, soy sauce, cornstarch, salt, and pepper. Pulse until the mixture is coarsely chopped.

4. Stuff the melon halves, place on a plate, drizzle with oyster sauce, if using this. Steam until the melons are tender and the stuffing cooked, about 20 to 25 minutes. Serve.

— *Bok Choy with Garlic* —

This is a quick, delicious, and nutritious vegetable dish. You may substitute any green leafy vegetable for the bok choy—including chard, spinach, mustard greens, Chinese broccoli, and oilseed rape—and still derive the same health benefits.

Good for: Anemia, diarrhea

Healing Properties: In Chinese as well as Western medicine, the vitamins and minerals in green leafy vegetables like bok choy act as a hearty tonic for the body. One reason is that chlorophyll—the substance that makes these vegetables green—acts as a blood builder and tissue renewer, thereby helping to bolster a weakened condition like anemia. Garlic, on the other hand, is very good for digestive problems, including diarrhea. Like other members of the onion family, garlic is extremely pungent and dispersing. It helps overcome stagnant qi and thereby can help balance the obstructive effect of overeating. From a Western perspective, both leafy green vegetables and garlic are considered antioxidants, which help guard against a myriad of diseases, including cardiovascular disease and cancer.

PREPARATION: 10 minutes   COOKING TIME: 5 to 7 minutes
SERVES: 2 to 4

---

1 bunch bok choy, about 1½ pounds
1 tablespoon soybean oil
3 garlic cloves, crushed
1 teaspoon salt
1 tablespoon water

1. Separate the bok choy leaves and wash well in cold water. Cut the leafy greens from the stems and cut the greens into ribbons. Set

aside. Slice the stems into sticks about ¼-inch thick and 2 inches long.

2. Heat the wok over medium high heat and add the oil. Stir-fry the crushed garlic cloves briefly, about 5 seconds, then add the bok choy stems. Stir-fry, tossing constantly, until the stems just begin to soften, about 5 minutes. Add the leaves and toss to mix well. Add the salt and water.

3. Reduce the heat, cover the wok, and steam 30 seconds to 1 minute. Serve.

— *Broccoli with Sesame Dressing* —

If you use the delicate Chinese broccoli with budded white flowers (gai lan), even children who hate broccoli will love this dish. Chinese broccoli is distinguished by its oval-shaped leaves, which have a bluish-green tint, and the white flowers in the middle of the plant. Use both leaves and stems, which you should peel if they seem woody. The dressing, which has a lovely sweet-sour flavor, makes a great topping for noodles, chicken, or salad.

Good for: Constipation, psoriasis

Healing Properties: Sesame oil is a cool, sweet food that has lubricating qualities. Taken internally, it can help relieve constipation and keep the skin moist (which may soothe the dryness and itchiness of psoriasis). You can even apply sesame oil directly onto the rash. From a Western perspective, broccoli is a wonderful source of roughage and thus can help keep your bowel movements regular. It also acts as a powerful antioxidant, which reduces the risks of disease and cancer.

PREPARATION: 10 minutes   COOKING TIME: 10 minutes   SERVES: 6

1 bunch broccoli, about 2 pounds
1 tablespoon salt

DRESSING
2 tablespoons sesame paste
3 tablespoons tepid water
2 tablespoons soy sauce
2 tablespoons sesame oil
2 tablespoons rice vinegar
1 teaspoon chili paste
1 teaspoon ground black pepper
2 teaspoons sugar
2 garlic cloves, finely minced

1. Bring a large pot of water to a boil.

2. Separate the florets from the broccoli stems. Peel the stems if they are woody.

3. Add the salt and the broccoli to the pot to blanch, stems first, then the florets, until the vegetable turns bright green. Drain immediately and plunge into ice water to cool completely. Drain and set aside.

4. To make the dressing, combine the sesame paste with the water in a small bowl. Stir until smooth and creamy. Whisk in the soy sauce, sesame oil, vinegar, chili paste, pepper, sugar, and garlic. Stir to blend well.

5. Dress the broccoli and serve at room temperature. Refrigerate any leftover dressing for future use.

— *Buddha's Delight with Dried Bean Curd Sticks* —

Buddha's Delight is a traditional Chinese vegetable dish that is both delectable and beautiful to look at. Serve over rice, if you like, or as a main dish on its own. It is often prepared in large amounts then put in the freezer for a special occasion like the New Year.

Good for: Anemia, insomnia

Healing Properties: Bean curd is a rich source of protein as well as iron, which helps alleviate anemia. Chinese dates also help bolster the blood by strengthening the spleen-pancreas. Dates also soothe nervousness, thus reducing insomnia. The other vegetables provide a host of essential vitamins and minerals.

PREPARATION: 30 minutes STANDING TIME: 20 minutes
COOKING TIME: 30 to 40 minutes SERVES: 8

---

4 ounces dried bean curd sticks
¼ cup tree ears
¼ cup lily buds
10 black mushrooms
1 ounce hair seaweed
2 tablespoons soybean oil
1 tablespoon minced ginger
1 cup sliced bamboo shoots
4 cups shredded Chinese cabbage (about 1 pound)
1 pound green daikon radish, peeled, cut in half, and sliced
20 red dates
3 tablespoons red nam yue
1 tablespoon dark soy sauce
2 cups water
½ teaspoon salt
1 teaspoon sugar
2 tablespoons sesame oil

1. Using separate bowls, soak the dried bean curd sticks, tree ears, and lily buds in hot water. In another bowl, soak the black mushrooms in 1 cup warm water. In another bowl, soak the hair seaweed in warm water and a little (only a few drops) of the vegetable oil. Let stand 15 to 20 minutes until all the ingredients are soft and pliable.

2. Drain and discard all the liquid, except for the mushroom water. Rinse the hair seaweed well to remove any grit. Set aside. Cut the bean curd sticks into pieces 3 to 4 inches long.

3. In a wok, heat the remaining oil and stir-fry the ginger until aromatic, about 10 seconds. Add the bean curd, tree ears, lily buds, mushrooms, bamboo shoots, cabbage, and daikon. Toss to blend well and add the nam yue, soy sauce, water, and the reserved mushroom water. Separate the hair seaweed as much as possible and add to the wok. Toss to blend well.

4. Reduce the heat and cook, covered, for 30 to 40 minutes, tossing occasionally, until the vegetables are soft and the flavor has penetrated throughout the mixture. Drizzle with sesame oil and serve.

— *Eggplant with Hot Bean Paste* —

This dish makes a filling main course for four or a side dish for six. Either way, its texture and flavor make it a perennial favorite. Try to make some extra and serve it cold as a relish at another meal.

Good for: Cold sores, hemorrhoids

Healing Properties: Eggplant is one of the most versatile medicinal foods in Chinese medicine. It is often used to treat bleeding problems, including bleeding hemorrhoids. Canker sores, too, are alleviated by eggplant. In Western medicine, eggplants are known to be a rich source of bioflavonoids, substances that help reduce the risk of heart disease and stroke.

PREPARATION: 15 minutes   STANDING TIME: 30 minutes
COOKING TIME: 15 minutes   SERVES: 4 to 6

4 Asian eggplants
1 tablespoon salt
1 tablespoon soybean oil
3 garlic cloves
1 tablespoon hot bean paste
1 tablespoon soy sauce
1 teaspoon sugar
½ cup water
2 teaspoons sesame oil

1. Wash the eggplants and cut them into 1-inch slices. Place them in a colander and sprinkle well with salt. Leave in the sink to drain 30 minutes. Rinse off all the salt and dry with paper towels.

2. Heat a wok until smoking, add the oil and garlic, and stir-fry until aromatic, about 10 seconds. Add the eggplant and toss to coat well. Add the hot bean paste, soy sauce, sugar, and water. Toss to mix, turn down the heat, and cook, stirring, until the eggplant is tender, about 15 minutes.

3. Remove from the heat and drizzle with sesame oil. Serve warm or chilled.

— *Kohlrabi with Swiss Chard Ribbons* —

You'll be pleasantly surprised at how good this dish looks and tastes—and the bonus is that it supplies a hearty dose of important vitamins and minerals with very little fat.

Good for: Diabetes, indigestion

Healing Properties: Kohlrabi is a pungent and bitter food that improves qi circulation throughout the body. It helps treat both indigestion and sugar imbalances, like diabetes and hypoglycemia.

PREPARATION: 10 minutes   COOKING TIME: 6 minutes
SERVES: 2 to 4

---

4 small kohlrabi, about 4 ounces each
1½ pounds Swiss chard
2 tablespoons soybean oil
2 garlic cloves, minced
1 teaspoon minced ginger
2 teaspoons cornstarch mixed with 1 tablespoon water
Salt and pepper to taste

1. Peel the thick skin from the kohlrabi and cut into matchstick-size pieces. Wash the chard well and separate the leaves from the stems. Discard the stems and cut the leaves into ribbons.

2. Heat the oil in a wok, add the garlic and ginger, and stir-fry until aromatic, about 10 seconds. Add the kohlrabi and stir-fry, tossing often, until tender, about 5 minutes. Add the chard ribbons and continue cooking until they wilt, about another minute. Add the cornstarch mixture, bring to a boil, and cook until the sauce thickens, about 1 minute. Season lightly with salt and pepper to taste and serve.

— *Steamed Pumpkin with Gingered Honey* —

When pumpkin is out of season, try using hubbard squash or sweet potatoes as substitutes in this recipe. The honey mixture is delicious on almost any vegetable.

Good for: Diabetes, colds and coughs, sinusitis

Healing Properties: In Chinese medicine, pumpkin is considered a warming, sweet food that benefits the spleen-pancreas and stomach. It is a mild diuretic as well. Ginger, on the other hand, induces perspiration, disperses cold, and affects the lungs, making it helpful in easing the congestion and fever associated with colds, coughs, and sinusitis.

PREPARATION: 10 minutes   COOKING TIME: 30 minutes   SERVES: 4

---

2 pounds pumpkin, cut into 2-inch cubes
½ cup honey
¼ teaspoon sesame oil
2 tablespoons slivered ginger
Sesame seeds, for garnish

1. Steam the pumpkin in a steamer basket until tender, about 30 minutes.
2. While the pumpkin is steaming, heat the honey with the sesame oil and ginger. Simmer gently over low heat until the honey is flavored, 5 to 10 minutes.
3. To serve, drizzle the warm honey over the pumpkin pieces. Garnish with sesame seeds, if desired.

— *Slivered Radish and Cilantro Salad* —

The fresh taste of cilantro works well in this refreshing salad, with a nifty bonus: it keeps your breath smelling sweet.

Good for: Bad breath, indigestion

Healing Properties: Cilantro (also known as Chinese parsley or coriander) is a refreshing herb that helps keep your breath fresh, as does the daikon radish. Both of these foods also reduce gastric acid and promote digestion, which may prevent indigestion from occurring.

PREPARATION: 10 minutes   SERVES: 4 to 6

---

1 large daikon radish, about 2 pounds
1 cup cilantro leaves, loosely packed
¼ cup rice vinegar
Salt to taste
¼ teaspoon cayenne pepper
2 teaspoons sugar

1. Peel the daikon radish and cut it into slivers about the size of matchsticks, or grate coarsely by hand. Toss the radish slivers and cilantro together lightly.

2. In a small bowl, combine the rice vinegar, salt, cayenne, and sugar. Stir to dissolve the sugar and mix well. Pour the dressing over the salad, toss to mix well, and serve.

— Silk Squash with Oyster Sauce —

This squash is what loofah sponges are made of, but you'd never know it in this savory, smooth dish. Silk squash are about ten to twelve inches long, dark green, and ridged. They have a subtle flavor and natural sweetness. Look for firm squash when you buy them.

Good for: Coughs and colds, chronic pain

Healing Properties: Squash is a warm, sweet food thought to heal inflammation and relieve pain. It also improves qi circulation. Silk squash is considered a winter squash, which means it contains even more vitamins (especially vitamin A) and minerals than summer squash.

PREPARATION: 10 minutes   COOKING TIME: 8 minutes   SERVES: 4

---

2 silk squash
1 tablespoon vegetable oil
2 slices ginger, about the size of a quarter
2 scallions, minced
¼ cup water chestnuts
2 tablespoons oyster sauce
1 teaspoon cornstarch mixed with 1 tablespoon water
Salt and pepper to taste

1. Peel the silk squash and cut them into pieces about 1-inch thick.
2. Heat a wok until it smokes; add the oil and ginger. Brown the ginger, then discard it. Add the scallions, silk squash, and water chestnuts. Stir-fry until the squash is tender, about 5 minutes. Add the oyster sauce and stir to blend. Add the cornstarch mixture and cook 1 minute or until the sauce thickens and coats the vegetables. Season to taste with salt and pepper. Serve.

— *Yam or Taro Root Braised with Nam Yue* —

This soothing, warm food helps relieve chronic pain while at the same time providing you with a host of essential vitamins and nutrients. Both yams and taro (another root vegetable) are especially rich in beta-carotene and vitamin C.

Good for: Chronic pain

Healing Properties: Both yams and taro strengthen the spleen-pancreas and promote qi energy. They also build the yin fluid capabilities of the kidneys, which in turn benefits dry and inflamed conditions in the body such as those that cause chronic pain.

PREPARATION: 10 minutes   COOKING TIME: 35 minutes
SERVES: 4 to 6 (as a side dish)

---

1 pound small taro roots, or yams
2 tablespoons soybean oil
1 tablespoon minced ginger
2 tablespoons nam yue
1 tablespoon soy sauce
1 teaspoon sugar
2 tablespoons white wine
1 cup water

1. Peel and cut the taros in half.
2. In a wok, heat the oil and stir-fry the ginger for about 10 seconds. Add the nam yue, soy sauce, sugar, and wine. Mash the nam yue and stir to blend.
3. Add the taro and water, bring to a boil, reduce the heat, cover, and simmer until the taro is soft, about 35 minutes. Serve.

⌞⌐⌐ *Fruit*

Fruit is generally eaten fresh by the Chinese but here is a traditional—and healthful—recipe that you will want to try.

— *Kumquats in Perfumed Syrup* —

These delicious kumquats keep well refrigerated and taste great by themselves or over ice cream. If you find this remedy works for you, prepare a batch before an airplane or boat ride and take it with you.

Good for: Indigestion, motion sickness, nausea

Healing Properties: Kumquats, believe it or not, are considered an excellent remedy for a host of digestive problems, including indigestion and nausea related to motion sickness.

PREPARATION: 20 minutes   COOKING TIME: 30 minutes
YIELD: 1½ cups

---

1 pound kumquats
3 cups water
1 cup sugar
6 star anise
6 cardamom seeds
2 teaspoons fennel seeds
1 teaspoon coriander seeds

1. Blanch the kumquats in a pot of boiling water for about 10 seconds. Let them cool and cut each fruit in half. Remove the seeds.

2. In a saucepan, combine the water and sugar. Add the star anise and the cardamom, fennel, and coriander seeds. Bring to a boil, reduce the heat, and cook, stirring once or twice, until the sugar is melted and the syrup is perfumed, about 10 to 15 minutes.

3. Add the fruit to the syrup and cook gently until the fruit is soft, about 30 minutes. Serve.

▣ Rice and Noodles

— Cellophane Noodles with Chinese Celery and Flowering White Cabbage —

Colorful and tasty, this noodle dish is sure to make "eating all your vegetables" a pleasurable activity. You can serve this hot over rice or cold as a salad.

Good for: Constipation, coughs, dizziness, hypertension

Healing Properties: Although it tastes cool and almost sweet, Chinese celery is considered a bitter food closely identified with the heart, where it clears excess heat and cleans the arteries. It is therefore very helpful in reducing high blood pressure and the dizziness that can accompany it. Flowering white cabbage is a delicate leafy vegetable unlike what most Americans think of as cabbage. The Chinese consider it to be helpful in treating constipation as well as stomach ulcers. From a Western standpoint, the carrots in this dish are an excellent source of beta-carotene, the precursor of vitamin A. A powerful antioxidant, beta-carotene protects against cancer and heart disease. It also acts as an anti-inflammatory on the mucous membranes, which helps to ease coughs.

PREPARATION: 25 minutes   STANDING TIME: 15 minutes
COOKING TIME: 15 minutes   SERVES: 6

---

8 ounces cellophane noodles (bean threads)
¼ cup tree ears
6 dried black mushrooms
½ pound flowering white cabbage (choi sum)
1 small bunch Chinese celery, about 1/2 pound
1 large carrot
2 tablespoons soybean oil
2 garlic cloves, minced
2 tablespoons dark soy sauce
1 tablespoon fermented bean curd (fu ye), *mashed*
½ cup vegetable broth
Salt and pepper, to taste
1 tablespoon sesame oil

1. In separate bowls, soak the cellophane noodles, tree ears, and mushrooms in warm water until soft, about 15 minutes. Drain, reserving the mushroom water. Remove the stems from the mushrooms and discard. Cut the mushroom caps if large.

2. Wash the flowering cabbage and celery well in cold water. Cut the vegetables into 2-inch pieces, keeping the cabbage stems and leaves separate. If the leaves are large, cut them into manageable pieces. Peel the carrot and cut it into matchstick-size pieces.

3. Heat a wok over high heat until smoking, add the oil and garlic, and stir-fry 10 seconds. Add the cabbage stems, celery, and carrots, stir-fry 1 minute, then add the mushrooms and tree ears. Toss to blend well, add 1 tablespoon of the soy sauce and the *fu ye,* and stir-fry until the vegetables are wilted, about 10 minutes. If the vegetables are dry, add 1 tablespoon of water. Remove the vegetables from the wok. Keep them warm.

4. Return the wok to the heat, and add the remaining soy sauce, broth, and the drained noodles. Season to taste with salt and pepper and mix well. Remove the noodles to a plate and top with the vegetable mix. Drizzle with the sesame oil and serve.

— Basic Congee —

Traditionally known as hsi-fan *, or "rice water," congee, or jook, is
a thin rice gruel often served at breakfast. It is so well liked,
though, people often eat it at lunch or for a late-night supper.
Although rice is the most common grain used to make congee,
millet, spelt, and other grains are sometimes used. The Chinese
believe that the longer you cook your congee, the more "powerful"
and healthful it becomes. If you have a crock-pot, use it to prepare
this dish—it will give you a superb congee without any risk of
burning.*

 *This basic recipe makes a congee that you can top with scal-
lions and ginger, a few peanuts, slices of fish or seafood, or any
cooked meats. It is also good just as it is, particularly if you are not
feeling well.*

Good for: Diarrhea, nausea

Healing Properties: This rice soup is highly digestible and tonifies the
blood and qi energy. Alone, it is good for harmonizing and calming
the digestive system, but you can add different ingredients for other
benefits.

PREPARATION: 5 minutes COOKING TIME: 2 hours (at least)
YIELD: 10 cups

½ cup long-grain rice
½ cup glutinous rice
16 cups cold water
½ teaspoon salt

1. In a crock-pot or heavy stockpot, combine the two kinds of
rice with the cold water and salt. Bring to a boil uncovered, then
reduce the heat to a low simmer, cover, and cook until a gruel is

formed, about 2 hours. If the congee is too thick, add water to get the consistency that you like. Serve.

— *Ginkgo Nut and Bean Curd Stick Congee* —

This version of congee can be served as either a sweet or savory dish. The recipe is a little different from our basic one, but either one will work with the ginkgo nuts and dried bean curd sticks. Traditionally, this dish is served as a late-night snack.

Good for: Diarrhea, hypertension, menopausal symptoms

Healing Properties: As discussed, congee with a rice base is helpful for a wide range of digestive problems. Bean curd, or tofu, is an exellent source of protein and helps to reduce heat signs, including those that accompany heart disease and hypertension. It also helps to build the yin, which the Chinese believe to be deficient in menopausal women.

PREPARATION: 10 minutes   COOKING TIME: 2 to 3 hours
SERVES: 12 or more

1½ cups long-grain rice
2 teaspoons vegetable oil, such as soy, safflower, canola
¼ teaspoon baking soda
16 cups water
8 ounces dried bean curd sticks
1 15-ounce can ginkgo nuts
Salt and pepper to taste (for a savory dish)
Sugar (to sprinkle on a sweet dish)

1. Rinse the rice and mix in the oil and baking soda. Add to a deep stockpot with 16 cups of water. Bring to a boil uncovered, then reduce the heat to a low simmer and cook, uncovered, for about 2 hours or until the congee has the consistency of a thin porridge. If it becomes too thick, add a little more water.

2. Meanwhile, rinse the bean curd sticks, soak them in warm water until soft, and cut into 3-inch-long pieces. Add the bean curd sticks to the congee about halfway through the cooking time.

3. When the congee is ready, add the drained ginkgo nuts and cook a few more minutes just until the nuts are warm.

4. Season with salt and pepper to taste for a savory dish, or sprinkle with sugar for a sweet one, and serve.

— Lo Mein with Mushrooms —

A perennial favorite in both Asian and American homes, this pasta dish with mushrooms is both nourishing and healing—and also very easy to make!

Good for: Colds, diarrhea

Healing Properties: The Chinese believe that most mushrooms, especially button mushrooms, help to ease diarrhea, as do lo mein noodles, which are made from wheat. Shiitake mushrooms are known to counteract high cholesterol levels and thus reduce the risk of arteriosclerosis and heart disease. Furthermore, they are said to be a natural source of interferon, a protein that appears to induce an immune response against viral infections, including the common cold.

PREPARATION: 15 minutes   COOKING TIME: 15 minutes   SERVES: 4

---

6 dried black mushrooms
8 ounces fresh shiitake mushrooms
10 ounces button mushrooms
1 tablespoon vegetable oil
2 tablespoons minced shallots
1 tablespoon minced garlic
2 tablespoons sherry
1 tablespoon mushroom soy sauce
1 teaspoon black pepper
1 teaspoon salt
2 tablespoons cream
1 pound fresh lo mein noodles
2 tablespoons chives, minced

1. In a bowl, soak the dried mushrooms in ½ cup warm water until soft, about 15 minutes. Drain, reserving the liquid. Remove and discard the stems. Cut the mushrooms into strips.

2. Meanwhile, clean the fresh mushrooms with damp paper towels. Cut into slices.

3. In a skillet, heat the oil and sauté the shallots and garlic about 1 minute. Add the mushrooms, sherry, mushroom soy sauce, pepper, salt, and reserved mushroom liquid. Simmer uncovered until most of the liquid is absorbed, about 10 minutes. Add the cream and cook another minute.

4. Bring a pot of water to a boil and cook the lo mein until tender, about 5 minutes. Drain and place on a serving platter.

5. Pour the mushrooms over the lo mein, toss to mix well, sprinkle with minced chives, and serve.

— *Soba Noodles with Mustard Greens* —

You can serve the noodles in the broth as a soup for an all-in-one meal or, as an alternative, serve them Japanese style—on the side, to be dipped into the broth. At the end of the meal, you can drink the flavorful broth. If you can't find Japanese pepper, you can substitute dried chili pepper flakes and ground black pepper.

Good for: Bronchitis, colds, flu

Healing Properties: Mustard greens have a warming nature and a pungent flavor that primarily influences the lungs. They help tonify and moisten the lungs and clear chest congestion, making them a perfect remedy for bronchitis. If you use chicken broth, this becomes a delicious chicken soup, which is a universal bromide for all kinds of upper respiratory tract infections.

PREPARATION: 10 minutes   COOKING TIME: 15 minutes
SERVES: 2 (as a main dish)

½ pound soba noodles
½ pound mustard greens (gai choy)
3 cups vegetable or chicken broth
2 tablespoons soy sauce
1 tablespoon sake
1 slice fresh ginger
1 scallion, minced
¼ teaspoon Japanese pepper (nanami togarashi)

1. Cook the soba noodles in boiling water until just done, about 5 minutes. Drain and refresh them with cold water. Wash the mustard greens well and cut into pieces.
2. Heat the broth, adding the soy sauce, sake, and ginger. Simmer 10 minutes or until the broth is flavored. Remove the ginger slice

and discard. Add the mustard greens and cook until the vegetable is wilted and tender, about 5 minutes.

3. If adding the noodles, stir them into the broth, sprinkle with the scallion and Japanese pepper, and serve in soup bowls. Or serve the broth in a bowl and the noodles sprinkled with scallion and pepper on the side. Dip the noodles into the broth, then eat. Drink the broth at the end of the meal.

— Brown Rice with Mung Bean Sprouts and Cabbage Ribbons —

Made with chicken stock, this brown rice and vegetable dish is both hearty and nutritious. The soy sauce and scallion give it just a little bite. Of course, you might want to add other herbs if you like a bit more flavor.

Good for: Candidiasis, constipation

Healing Properties: Mung bean sprouts are good for reducing yeast overgrowth (candidiasis). Very cooling with a sweet flavor, they also help to detoxify the body of impurities of all kinds. Chinese cabbage is also cooling and sweet, and helps to moisten the intestines and treat constipation.

PREPARATION: 15 minutes   COOKING TIME: 45 minutes
SERVES: 4 to 6

---

2 cups brown rice
4 cups low-sodium chicken broth
1 scallion, green and white parts, minced
2 cups (¼ pound) mung bean sprouts
2 cups (½ pound) Chinese cabbage, shredded into ribbons
1½ teaspoons thin soy sauce
1 teaspoon black pepper

1. In a saucepan, combine the brown rice with the broth. Bring to a boil, reduce the heat, and cook, covered, until the rice is cooked through, about 45 minutes.

2. Stir in the scallion, mung bean sprouts, cabbage ribbons, soy sauce, and pepper. Mix well. Steam another 5 minutes. Serve.

— *Coconut Sweet Rice* —

This rich-tasting rice is good eaten with a spicy stew or curry, but can also be sweetened and used as a dessert, especially if you top it with fresh papaya or mango. If you wish to make a sweet dish, skip the salt and add sugar to the coconut milk instead. Make sure to stir until all the sugar dissolves before adding the rice. Please note: Coconut milk is high in saturated fat, so if you're concerned with your weight, or if you eat lots of meats and nuts on a regular basis, limit how often you indulge in this dish!

Good for: Edema, urinary infections

Healing Properties: Coconut milk is a slightly sweet and aromatic food in Chinese medicine. It helps produce fluids, promotes urination, and destroys intestinal parasites.

PREPARATION: 5 minutes   COOKING TIME: 20 minutes
STANDING TIME: 5 minutes   SERVES: 4 to 6

---

1 cup sweet rice
Pinch of salt (or sugar if using as a dessert)
2 cups coconut milk

1. Rinse the rice in one or two changes of cold water.

2. If you're making a savory rice to serve with meats or a curry, place the rice in a deep saucepan, add a pinch of salt and the coconut milk, then bring to a boil. Immediately turn the heat down and con-

tinue cooking, uncovered, until nearly all the coconut milk is absorbed and a layer of cream remains. Stir the rice, cover, and let sit 5 minutes.

3. If you're making a sweet rice, place the coconut milk in the pan with sugar to taste and stir until all the sugar dissolves. Then add the rice and cook as directed in step 2.

⊡ Meat

— Hoisin Beef with Red and Green Peppers —

Spicy but not overly hot, this beef dish makes a colorful entrée for meat lovers. You can find hoisin sauce, which is made with soybeans and wheat flour, in Asian markets and most supermarkets. You'll probably have lots of sauce left over, which you can use as a marinade for chicken and fish.

Good for: Anemia, urinary infections

Healing Properties: The red and green peppers in this dish are hot, pungent foods that warm the intestines, promote digestion and urination, and thus help to clear the urinary tract of impurities. Beef, on the other hand, is a warming sweet food that strengthens the stomach and spleen and fortifies the blood, thereby reversing anemia. That's true from a Western perspective as well, as beef contains the iron that many people with anemia lack in their diets.

PREPARATION: 15 minutes   COOKING TIME: 15 minutes   SERVES: 4

---

1 pound filet mignon, cut into 1-inch cubes
2 tablespoons dark soy sauce
2 teaspoons brandy
1 tablespoon cornstarch
¼ cup hoisin sauce
1 tablespoon sesame oil
¼ cup water
2 tablespoons soybean oil
2 garlic cloves, minced
2 teaspoons ginger, minced
1 tablespoon scallion, minced (white part only)
1 red pepper, trimmed, seeded, and cut into 1-inch squares
1 green pepper, trimmed, seeded, and cut into 1-inch squares

1. In a small bowl, combine the meat, 1 tablespoon of the soy sauce, brandy, and cornstarch. Toss to coat the meat well. In another bowl, combine the hoisin sauce, sesame oil, and water.

2. Heat a wok until just smoking, add the oil, and swirl to coat the sides of the wok well. Add the garlic, ginger, and scallion. Stir-fry until aromatic, about 10 seconds.

3. In batches, add the meat and stir-fry until it is seared but still pink in the middle, about 5 to 7 minutes. Remove to a plate and keep warm.

4. Return the wok to the heat and stir-fry the peppers, tossing frequently, about 1 minute. Add the meat and toss to heat through.

5. Stir the hoisin mixture and add it to the wok. Stir-fry another minute, tossing to blend well, and serve.

— Soybean Sprouts with Beef —

Although this is a very traditional way of serving soy sprouts, you can make this a vegetarian dish by leaving out the beef and still derive the same health benefits. In fact, the soybean is called the beef of China because of its high protein content and essential fatty acids. Best of all, it contains no saturated fat or cholesterol.

Good for: Arthritis

Healing Properties: Soybean sprouts are cooling with a sweet flavor; they also act as a diuretic that can help relieve the aches and pains associated with arthritis.

PREPARATION: 5 minutes   COOKING TIME: 6 minutes   SERVES: 2

¼ pound beef flank
1 teaspoon cornstarch
1 tablespoon plus 1 teaspoon soy sauce

1 teaspoon minced ginger
1 teaspoon rice wine
2 tablespoons soybean oil
½ pound soybean sprouts
Salt and pepper to taste

1. Slice the beef flank into pieces about ¼-inch wide and 1-inch long.

2. In a bowl, combine the beef with the cornstarch, 1 teaspoon of the soy sauce, ginger, and wine.

3. Heat the wok and add the oil. Stir-fry the beef until it loses its pink color, about 5 minutes. Add the soybean sprouts, the remaining soy sauce, and 1 tablespoon water. Stir-fry, tossing, until the sprouts just wilt, about 1 minute. Season with salt and pepper to taste and serve.

— Spicy Lamb with Wide Rice Noodles —

Fresh rice noodles, called ho fun *in China, are available in Asian stores. The lamb tastes just as good served with dried rice noodles (rice vermicelli or* mei fun*), which are available in most supermarkets. In this recipe, the noodles are eaten at room temperature. If you would like to serve the dish hot, heat the noodles, covered, in the oven.*

Good for: Nausea, urinary problems

Healing Properties: Rice noodles help relieve nausea, and lamb strengthens kidney deficiencies, which can help reduce urinary problems such as incontinence.

PREPARATION: 20 minutes   COOKING TIME: 5 minutes
SERVES: 4 to 6

¾ pound fresh rice noodle sheets
2 teaspoons light soy sauce
1 tablespoon sesame oil
1 tablespoon peanut oil
2 garlic cloves, minced
1 teaspoon dry red chili flakes
½ pound lean ground lamb
2 tablespoons yellow bean sauce
¼ cup chicken stock
Pinch of sugar
2 scallions, minced

1. Cut the rice noodle sheets into wide ribbons. Toss with the soy sauce and sesame oil and place on a serving platter.

2. Heat a wok until smoking, add the peanut oil, and stir-fry the garlic and red chili flakes for about 10 seconds. Add the lamb and cook, breaking up the meat, until it loses its pink color, about 5 minutes. Add the bean paste, stock, and sugar. Bring the mixture to a boil and cook, stirring, another 1 to 2 minutes.

3. Spoon the lamb mixture over the noodles. Sprinkle with scallions and serve.

— *Pork Liver with Garlic Chive Flowers* —

The Chinese consider pork liver superior to beef or calves' liver, in both taste and medicinal qualities. However, calves' liver will work almost as well in this recipe, and it may be easier to find.

Good for: Anemia, diabetes

Healing Properties: In the diet, liver of all types builds the blood and strengthens the liver, making it especially healthful for those who suffer from anemia. Pork liver in particular works to strengthen the spleen and pancreas, which helps to alleviate diabetes.

PREPARATION: 10 minutes   COOKING TIME: 3 minutes   SERVES: 4

---

1 pound pork liver
6 ounces garlic chive flowers
2 teaspoons thin soy sauce
1 tablespoon oyster sauce
½ teaspoon pepper
2 tablespoons soybean oil

1. Trim the liver and cut into thin slices. Cut the chive flowers into 2-inch-long pieces.

2. In a small bowl, combine the soy sauce, oyster sauce, and pepper with 2 tablespoons water.

3. Heat a wok until smoking, add the oil and the liver, tossing rapidly. Immediately add the flowers and mix well, then add the sauce mixture, tossing constantly. Blend well. The liver will cook in 3 to 5 minutes and the chive flowers wilt. Do not overcook. Serve.

— *Braised Pork with Black Bean Sauce* —

This is a dish that tastes even more delicious if you prepare it a day before serving. This provides extra time for the flavors to mingle, and also allows you to remove any fat that rises to the surface as it cools.

Good for: Hepatitis

Healing Properties: Pork helps to bolster the liver, which is the primary organ involved in hepatitis.

PREPARATION: 15 minutes   COOKING TIME: 1 hour   SERVES: 6

2 ½ pounds boneless pork ribs
2 tablespoons fermented black beans
2 tablepoons soybean oil
3 cloves garlic, minced
2 slices fresh ginger
2 scallions, minced
⅓ cup dark soy sauce
2 tablespoons oyster sauce
2 tablespoons brown sugar
1 teaspoon black pepper
1 cup water

1. Trim any excess fat from the pork. Cut the meat into 1-inch cubes. Rinse the black beans and mash slightly.
2. In a saucepan or wok, heat the oil and brown the pork in batches. Remove to a plate.
3. Add the garlic, ginger, scallions, and black beans. Stir-fry until aromatic, about 10 seconds. Add the soy sauce, oyster sauce, brown sugar, and pepper. Bring to a simmer and return the pork to the pan. Add the water and cook until the pork is tender, about 45 minutes. Serve.

— *Five-Spice Pork with Nam Yue* —

This dish is tasty and rich. Use any leftover pork for stir-fried rice or add it to vegetables for a bit of protein. Nam yue is bean curd pickled in rice wine. It adds a distinctive flavor to this pork dish.

Good for: Chronic fatigue, diabetes, sinusitis

Healing Properties: The five-spice powder helps to relieve the pain and congestion of sinusitis, while the pork strengthens the kidneys, spleen-pancreas, and stomach.

PREPARATION: 10 minutes   STANDING TIME: 5 hours or overnight
COOKING TIME: 35 minutes   SERVES: 6 to 8

---

3 pounds pork butt, with some fat
2 tablespoons hoisin sauce
1 tablespoon soy sauce
1 teaspoon five-spice powder
1 tablespoon nam yue
3 tablespoons maltose

1. Cut the pork into strips about 3 inches thick.
2. In a bowl combine the hoisin sauce, soy sauce, five-spice powder, nam yue, and maltose. Spread the sauce over the pork strips, cover, and refrigerate at least 5 hours or overnight.
3. Preheat the oven to 350 degrees F. Place the pork strips on a rack and roast for 25 to 30 minutes until tender.
4. Preheat the broiler and char the pork 5 minutes until it is brown at the edges, or barbecue the pork on a charcoal grill outdoors. Serve.

⊡ Fish and Seafood

— Steamed Carp on Mustard Greens —

The combination of fish and leafy greens is a healthy one from both an Eastern and a Western perspective, and the flavorful oils and ginger give the dish a unique and delicate flavor. Although carp is the preferred fish from a Chinese medicine standpoint, you can substitute sea bass or snapper if you cannot find carp.

To steam the fish, you will need a ten-inch plate and a twelve- to fourteen-inch bamboo steamer basket with lid.

Good for: Cough, flu

Healing Properties: Carp is a neutral, sweet food that facilitates water passage—relieving congestion—and acts on the spleen and kidneys. Interestingly enough, carp is also known to help increase lactation: a bonus for nursing mothers!

PREPARATION: 20 minutes   COOKING TIME: 30 to 40 minutes
SERVES: 4 to 6

---

1 fresh carp, with head and tail, 9 to 12 inches long
¼ cup ginger, slivered
¼ cup scallion, slivered
1 tablespoon soy sauce
2 teaspoons sesame oil
1 tablespoon peanut oil
1 garlic clove, mashed
3 to 4 cups mustard greens, cleaned
½ teaspoon salt

1. Have the fish gutted and scaled at the market. Rinse and pat dry.

2. Make three slits on the top side of the fish and lay it on a 10-inch plate. Spread the ginger and scallion over the fish and drizzle with the soy sauce and sesame oil. Place the plate in the steamer basket and put it in a wok filled with enough water to touch the bottom of the steamer basket. Steam the fish until firm to the touch, about 30 to 40 minutes. Do not let the wok steam dry or the basket will burn. Replenish the water periodically.

3. While the fish is cooking, heat another wok until smoking, add the peanut oil and garlic, cook until the garlic browns, then discard it. Add the mustard greens and stir-fry until wilted. Sprinkle them with salt and lay on a serving platter.

4. Carefully transfer the fish onto the greens, pour over any juices that have accumulated, and serve.

— *Clams and Mussels in Black Bean Sauce* —

The textures and tastes of this dish make it a truly interesting and savory main course. The black beans transform this recipe from an ordinary seafood dish to a sublime taste treat.

Good for: Edema, hemorrhoids

Healing Properties: Both clams and mussels nurture the yin and moisten dryness, making them perfect tonics to help facilitate proper fluid distribution. They also help ease the swelling of hemorrhoids.

PREPARATION: 30 minutes   COOKING TIME: 10 to 15 minutes
SERVES: 4

2 dozen clams
2 dozen mussels
2 tablespoons fermented black beans
2 garlic cloves, minced
1 tablespoon minced ginger
2 tablespoons soybean oil
⅓ cup dry white wine
2 scallions, green parts only, minced

1. With a stiff brush, clean the clams and mussels under cold running water. Be sure to pull off any "beards" protruding from the mussels. Drain well.

2. Rinse the black beans under cold water and mash coarsely together with the garlic, ginger, and ½ tablespoon of the oil.

3. Heat a wok until just smoking. Add the remaining oil and stir-fry the black bean mixture until aromatic, about 10 seconds. Add the clams and toss to blend. Cover and cook 30 seconds, then add the mussels and toss well. Add the wine, cover, and cook until the mussels and clams have opened.

4. Remove to a serving platter, discarding any unopened shellfish. Pour all the sauce over the shellfish, and sprinkle with scallion to serve.

— Fish-Filled Wontons —

These wontons are good in soup, with vegetables, or for a special treat, deep-fried for a delicious appetizer.

Good for: Cold sores, indigestion

Healing Properties: Water chestnuts are the key ingredient here as far as canker sores are concerned. Some Chinese medicine practitioners even prescribe chewing plain water chestnuts slowly or drinking water chestnut juice to soothe mouth sores. White fish like flounder are considered neutral sweet foods that help to promote proper body fluid distribution. Their strengthening action on spleen-pancreas function helps to treat indigestion and improve the appetite.

PREPARATION: 30 minutes   YIELD: About 60

½ pound flounder fillets
8 water chestnuts
1 scallion, minced
1 teaspoon ginger, minced
1 tablespoon thin soy sauce
½ teaspoon salt
½ teaspoon pepper
2 teaspoons cornstarch
2 teaspoons sesame oil
1 package wonton wrappers
1 egg beaten with 1 tablespoon water

1. In a food processor, combine the fish, water chestnuts, scallion, ginger, soy sauce, salt, pepper, cornstarch, and sesame oil. Process until the mixture forms a smooth blend.

2. Lay the wonton wrappers on the work surface, several at a time. Spoon a scant teaspoon of the filling onto the center of each wrapper. Brush the edges with the egg mixture, fold over corner to corner to form a triangle, and join two corners of the triangle, to form a peaked cap. Continue until all the filling is used up.

3. Place the finished wontons on a well-floured cookie sheet.

4. Boil the wontons in a soup, then sauté them in a little olive oil; or, if calories and fat content are not a concern, they can be deep-fried.

— *Fish with Lemon Sauce* —

In traditional Chinese cooking, this dish would be deep-fried. Here, though, we've created a delicious version using only 4 tablespoons of oil so you can enjoy the flavors and not miss the fat.

Good for: Colds, hypertension, indigestion

Healing Properties: As is true in Western medicine, lemon and other citrus fruits are excellent for easing cold symptoms. In Chinese medicine, lemons have a cooling, astringent flavor with antiseptic, antimicrobial, and mucus-resolving action. They also help to cleanse the blood and reduce high blood pressure. Both white fish and lemon also soothe the digestive tract.

PREPARATION: 20 minutes   COOKING TIME: 15 minutes   SERVES: 6

2 pounds cod fillets
¼ cup flour
¼ cup cornstarch
1 teaspoon salt
½ teaspoon pepper
4 teapoons peanut oil

SAUCE
1 tablespoon soybean oil
1 teaspoon ginger, minced
2 tablespoons grated lemon zest
¼ cup lemon juice
½ cup chicken stock or water
1 teaspoon thin soy sauce
1 teaspoon sugar
2 teaspoons sesame oil
1 teaspoon cornstarch

1. Remove any bones from the cod fillets. Cut them into 2-inch-square pieces and pat dry with paper towels.

2. Sift together the flour, cornstarch, salt, and pepper. Spread out the mixture on a piece of wax paper. Coat the fish well with it.

3. Heat the peanut oil in a wok until just smoking and fry the fish pieces, turning once to brown on both sides. Remove to paper towels to drain. Keep warm.

4. In a small saucepan, heat the soybean oil and cook the minced ginger for a few seconds. Add the lemon zest, lemon juice, stock, soy sauce, sugar, and sesame oil. Mix the cornstarch with 1 tablespoon cold water. Add to the sauce and bring to a boil. Cook 1 minute or until the sauce thickens.

5. Return the fish to a platter and pour the sauce over the fish to serve.

— Fish Poached with Rice Wine Sauce —

Cooking fish in this way makes it delicate and moist. Be sure to place the fish in a single layer and cover completely with boiling water to avoid overcooking and drying it out.

Good for: Arthritis, stomachache

Healing Properties: The fennel seeds in this recipe help to relieve the pain of arthritis, as well as soothe a stomachache. Fennel seeds also promote energy circulation and affect the kidneys, bladder, and stomach.

PREPARATION: 10 minutes   COOKING TIME: 15 minutes
SERVES: 6

2 pounds firm white fish fillets, about 1-inch thick
1 cup cornstarch
1 cup bottled clam juice
1 cup vegetable or chicken stock
¼ cup rice wine
2 tablespoons thin soy sauce
3 tablespoons rice vinegar
2 teaspoons fennel seeds
1 teaspoon sugar
1 tablespoon sesame oil
1 tablespoon cornstarch mixed with 2 tablespoons cold water
¼ cup slivered ginger
¼ cup slivered scallion
Freshly ground black pepper
2 tablespoons vegetable oil

1. Remove any bones from the fish and cut it into 3-inch-square pieces. Coat the fish pieces with cornstarch. Place in a single layer in a shallow baking pan. Bring 10 cups of water to a rolling boil and pour over the fish. Immediately cover the baking pan with tinfoil. The fish will cook as the water cools. Let stand at least 10 minutes.

2. In a saucepan, combine the clam juice, stock, wine, soy sauce, vinegar, fennel seeds, sugar, and sesame oil. Bring to a boil and simmer 5 minutes. Add the cornstarch mixture and cook until the sauce thickens. Keep warm.

3. With a slotted spoon, remove the fish to a serving platter. Sprinkle with ginger, scallions, and black pepper.

4. Heat the oil in a small saucepan until smoking and immediately pour over the fish. The oil will sizzle. Pour sauce over fish. Serve.

— Mussels Steamed in Rice Wine —

*The basic broth in this recipe can be used for steaming clams, too.
Be sure to serve some of the broth with the mussels—it's delicious.
If any broth remains, save it to add to another fish dish you pre-
pare in the future.*

Good for: Menstrual problems

Healing Properties: Clams and mussels are cooling, salty foods that
moisten dryness and facilitate proper body fluid movement, which
helps reduce the bloating and cramping that often occur just before
a woman gets her period.

PREPARATION: 10 minutes   COOKING TIME: 15 to 20 minutes
SERVES: 4

---

2 pounds mussels
2 cups clam juice
1 cup rice wine
3 tablespoons sweet butter
¼ cup minced shallots
1 teaspoon minced ginger
2 scallions, minced
1 tablespoon minced fresh thyme
4 tablespoons minced parsley

1. Wash the mussels under cold water with a stiff brush. Pull off
any "beards." Drain the mussels in a colander.

2. In a pot large enough to hold the mussels, combine the clam
juice, rice wine, butter, shallots, ginger, scallions, and thyme. Bring
to a simmer and cook, covered, until the liquid is flavored, about 10
minutes.

3. Add the mussels to the liquid and cook, covered, stirring occasionally. Remove the mussels as they open. Do not overcook.

4. Sprinkle the mussels with parsley and serve with a little of the
broth.

— *Oyster, Mushroom, and Bean Curd Stew* —

This savory vegetable-and-oyster stew is sure to help calm your nerves, ease any intestinal problems you might have, and taste delicious all at the same time.

Good for: Diarrhea, insomnia

Healing Properties: Mushrooms are often used as a remedy for diarrhea, and oysters are known to calm nervousness and nurture the quieter yin energy, thereby making it easier to fall asleep. Both will help to bolster your immune system, thereby protecting you from infection.

PREPARATION: 20 minutes   STANDING TIME: 15 minutes
COOKING TIME: 22 minutes   SERVES: 6

---

6 large dried Chinese mushrooms
¼ cup tree ears
1 pound firm bean curd (tofu)
¼ cup dark soy sauce
2 tablespoons oyster sauce
¼ cup white wine
1 star anise
2 slices ginger
2 teaspoons cornstarch mixed with 2 tablespoons cold water
3 scallions, cut into 2-inch pieces
1 pint shucked oysters

1. In a small bowl, soak the mushrooms in 1½ cups warm water. In another bowl, soak the tree ears in warm water. Let them stand 15 minutes. Drain the mushrooms, reserving the water. Remove the stems and discard. Cut the mushrooms in quarters. Drain the tree ears, rinse them in cold water if gritty, and set aside. Cut the bean curd into 2-inch squares.

2. In a saucepan, combine the reserved mushroom water, soy

sauce, oyster sauce, white wine, star anise, and ginger. Bring to a boil, reduce the heat, and add the mushrooms, tree ears, and bean curd. Simmer 20 minutes. Add the cornstarch mixture, return to the boil, and simmer until the sauce thickens slightly, about 1 minute.

3. Add the scallions and oysters and cook until the oysters are just done, about 1 to 2 minutes. Serve.

— Oysters Steamed in Egg Custard —

Be sure to use a flat dish to steam the custard, otherwise it will take too long to set. Never let the water come to a rolling boil, as air bubbles will form and your custard will be spongy.

Good for: Diarrhea, indigestion, insomnia

Healing Properties: Both the eggs and the oysters help soothe an upset stomach and alleviate diarrhea. As for insomnia, oysters are known to be especially useful for conditions involving deficiencies of yin like insomnia.

PREPARATION: 15 minutes   COOKING TIME: 20 minutes
SERVES: 4 to 6

---

1 pint shucked oysters
6 eggs
2 teaspoons thin soy sauce
½ teaspoon white pepper
1 teaspoon salt
1 teaspoon sesame oil
1 scallion, green and white parts, minced

1. Drain the oysters well, reserving 3 tablespoons of the juice.
2. In a bowl, stir the eggs with the oyster juice to blend well. Do not beat the eggs with a fork, as no foam should form. Add the soy sauce, pepper, and salt. Stir well.

3. Grease a heatproof pie dish with the sesame oil and pour in the egg mixture. Arrange the oysters evenly in the egg mixture and sprinkle with the scallions. Set the dish in a bamboo steamer basket with a lid. Cover and steam over low heat 15 to 20 minutes or until the eggs are lightly set and the oysters are just cooked. Serve.

— *Scallops with Long Beans* —

This dish makes a hearty main course for four to six people. Serve with white or brown rice if you'd like a little starch in your meal. These long beans are really from the black-eyed pea family. They stay firm even if slightly overcooked.

Good for: Candidiasis

Healing Properties: Beans help energize the spleen and kidney and therefore can be helpful in alleviating yeast infections. An added benefit is that scallops are among the most nutritious and least fatty of all seafood.

PREPARATION: 10 minutes   COOKING TIME: 14 minutes
SERVES: 4 to 6

---

1 bunch long beans (about 1 ½ pounds)
1 tablespoon salt (or to taste)
½ pound bay scallops
1 tablespoon peanut oil
1 tablespoon sesame oil
1 tablespoon garlic, minced
1 teaspoon pepper
2 tablespoons black sesame seeds

1. Bring a pot of water to a boil.
2. Rinse the beans and cut into 2-inch pieces.
3. Add the beans and salt to the water and blanch until just ten-

der, 3 to 5 minutes. Drain and plunge into ice water. Drain well cold. Set aside.

4. Remove the muscles from the scallops, if desired.

5. Heat a wok until just smoking, add the two oils and the minced garlic, stir once, then add the blanched beans.

6. Cook, tossing, until the beans are warm, about 3 minutes.

7. Add the scallops and pepper, and stir-fry until the scallops turn white, about 1 minute.

8. Remove from the heat and sprinkle with black sesame seeds to serve.

— *Shrimp Wrapped in Seaweed* —

Traditionally, this is a deep-fried dish, but in the interest of healthier eating, this recipe calls for sautéeing the shrimp in just two tablespoons of oil. It tastes just as crisp and delicious. Use a nonstick skillet if possible.

Good for: Bronchitis, flu

Healing Properties: The nori, or seaweed, in this dish is often used to treat chronic bronchitis. You may also want to add extra ginger, which helps to relieve congestion. From a Western standpoint, the shrimp is an excellent source of low-fat protein.

PREPARATION: 15 minutes STANDING TIME: 2 hours or longer
COOKING TIME: 2 to 3 minutes SERVES: 4 (as an appetizer)

---

8 large shrimp
1 tablespoon thin soy sauce
1 teaspoon minced ginger
1 tablespoon sherry
¼ teaspoon black pepper
¼ cup cornstarch
1 sheet nori, 7½ by 8 inches
2 tablespoons peanut oil

1. Peel the shrimp, leaving on the tails, and devein them. In a bowl, combine the soy sauce, ginger, sherry, and pepper. Add the shrimp and toss to coat well. Marinate for 2 hours or longer in the refrigerator.

2. Sprinkle cornstarch onto a plate or wax paper. Remove the shrimp from the marinade and coat with cornstarch. The shrimp will remain slightly wet.

3. Cut the nori sheet into eight strips and then cut each strip in half. Wrap a piece of nori around each shrimp, leaving the tail exposed. Seal the nori with a little water.

4. In an 8-inch nonstick skillet, heat the oil. Add the shrimp in two or three batches without crowding and sauté until the tails turn pink and the shrimp are crisp. Turn the shrimp and cook on the other side until they are firm to the touch, about 3 to 5 minutes. Remove and drain on paper towels. Serve hot.

— *Squid with Thin Wheat Noodles in Spicy Sauce* —

If you cannot find fresh red hot chilis, use the dried ones and crumble them. A little diced sweet red pepper makes a nice garnish.

Good for: Candidiasis, colds, flu

Healing Properties: The most pungent onion family member, garlic inhibits the common cold virus and other microorganisms associated with disease. Garlic also helps to eliminate toxins from the body.

PREPARATION: 20 minutes   COOKING TIME: 15 minutes
SERVES: 4 to 6

2 pounds squid
1 pound fresh thin wheat noodles
3 tablespoons vegetable oil
4 garlic cloves, sliced
2 tablespoons shallots
1 teaspoon minced ginger
3 red hot chilis
¼ cup dry white wine
2 teaspoons salt (or to taste)
1 teaspoon pepper
½ cup cilantro leaves, loosely packed

1. Clean the squid and cut into rings. Bring a pot of water to the boil and cook the noodles until just done, about 3 to 5 minutes. Drain.

2. In the meantime, heat the oil in a deep saucepan or wok and stir-fry the garlic, shallots, and ginger briefly; add the chilis and stir to mix.

3. Add the wine, salt, and pepper, and simmer 1 minute. Add the squid and cook until the squid just turns white.

4. Remove from the heat, add the noodles and cilantro leaves, and toss to mix well. Serve at once.

▣ Poultry

— Steamed Chicken "Cake" —

This dish is traditionally made with ground pork, but chicken is lower in fat, and best of all, it tastes just as good. If you prefer, you can prepare this dish as you would a meatloaf and bake it in the oven.

Good for: Cold sores, diabetes

Healing Properties: Practitioners of Chinese medicine often suggest water chestnuts and snow peas to treat cold sores. A warming, sweet food, chicken is often used in Chinese medicine to correct spleen-pancreas imbalances like diabetes.

PREPARATION: 15 minutes   COOKING TIME: 30 to 35 minutes
SERVES: 4

---

1 tablespoon tree ears
6 water chestnuts
¼ cup snow peas
1 pound ground chicken
1 teaspoon minced ginger
2 teaspoons thin soy sauce
2 tablespoons chicken stock
1 tablespoon cornstarch
½ teaspoon salt
½ teaspoon pepper
2 teaspoons sesame oil

1. In a small bowl, soak the tree ears in warm water until soft, about 10 to 15 minutes. Drain and rinse if gritty, and coarsely chop them.

2. Coarsely chop the water chestnuts and combine with the tree ears.

3. Bring a small saucepan of water to the boil, blanch the snow peas a few seconds, or until they turn bright green. Drain immediately and plunge into ice water. When cold, drain and coarsely chop the snow peas and combine them with the tree ears and water chestnuts.

4. In another bowl, mix together the ground chicken, ginger, soy sauce, stock, cornstarch, salt, and pepper. Blend well, then mix in the vegetable mixture, tossing to blend.

5. Lightly oil a heatproof bowl with 1 teaspoon of sesame oil. Press the chicken mixture into the bowl and place it in a steamer basket over water. Cover and steam 30 to 35 minutes, until the juices run clear and the chicken "cake" is firm to the touch. Drizzle with the remaining sesame oil and serve.

— Chicken Cubes with Lichee and Plum Sauce —

The sweetness of the plum sauce with the lichee nuts create an interesting combination of textures and flavors.

Good for: Cold sores, diabetes, menstrual problems, chronic pain

Healing Properties: Plums, especially cooked plums, help to relieve cold sores and mouth cankers. In fact, they are known to ease all kinds of pain—including emotional upset. Practitioners of Chinese medicine also prescribe plums to treat liver disease, especially cirrhosis of the liver. Chicken helps restore pancreatic imbalances such as those that cause diabetes. Lichees help relieve pain of all kinds, including menstrual cramps.

PREPARATION: 10 minutes   COOKING TIME: 6 minutes   SERVES: 4

1 pound skinless, boneless chicken breasts
2 teaspoons cornstarch
1 egg white
2 teaspoons thin soy sauce
1 teaspoon water
¼ teaspoon ground pepper
2 cups lichees, canned
½ cup lichee juice, reserved from lichees
2 tablespoons soybean oil
2 teaspoons minced ginger
½ cup plum sauce (duck sauce)
⅓ cup chicken stock or water
½ cup water chestnuts
1 scallion, white and green parts, minced

1. Cut the chicken into ½-inch cubes.

2. In a small bowl, combine the chicken, cornstarch, egg white, soy sauce, water, and pepper. Drain the lichees and reserve ½ cup of the juice. Set aside.

3. Heat a wok until just smoking, add the oil and ginger, then stir-fry until aromatic, about 10 seconds. Add the chicken and cook until it turns white, about 5 minutes. Toss often.

4. Add the plum sauce, lichee juice, lichees, chicken stock, and water chestnuts.

5. Toss to blend well, and cook until the stock thickens slightly and the ingredients are heated through. Sprinkle with scallions and serve.

— *Chicken Legs with Pineapple and Mandarin Peel* —

You can prepare this dish a day ahead, and then chill it and remove any fat, although since skinless chicken is used very little fat actually remains. The dish will keep several days refrigerated and can be reheated in the microwave. The more time the flavors have to mingle and merge, the better the dish tastes.

Good for: Flatulence

Healing Properties: Pineapple is a neutral, sweet-sour food that contains the enzyme bromelain, which increases the ability of the intestines to digest food. And the more efficiently you digest food, the less chance you'll have to suffer from flatulence. Eaten on its own, pineapple is a delicious thirst quencher.

PREPARATION: 20 minutes   STANDING TIME: 10 minutes
COOKING TIME: 45 minutes   SERVES: 4

---

8 chicken legs or 4 legs with thighs, about 2 ½ pounds, skin removed
1 fresh pineapple
4 pieces dried mandarin peel
2 teaspoons vegetable oil
¼ cup sherry
¼ cup dark soy sauce
2 cups homemade chicken stock or low-sodium, canned chicken stock
1 cinnamon stick
4 star anise
2 slices fresh ginger
1 teaspoon sugar

1. Clean the chicken; separate the thighs from the legs if using whole legs.

2. Pare the pineapple, core it, and cut it into chunks. You will have about 4 cups. Reserve any juices that run off.

3. In a small bowl, soak the dried mandarin peel in water until soft, about 10 minutes. Drain, reserving the water, and cut into slivers.

4. Heat a wok or a deep saucepan, add the oil, and lightly brown the chicken pieces. Add the sherry and cook 5 minutes. Then add the soy sauce, stock, reserved mandarin water, mandarin peel, cinnamon, star anise, ginger, and sugar. Bring to a boil, reduce the heat, and simmer 10 minutes. Add the pineapple chunks and continue cooking until the chicken is tender and the juices run clear when the legs are pricked, about 20 minutes.

— Chicken with Walnuts —

This flavorful dish is quick to prepare and very healthful. Serve it with rice and a side of your favorite vegetables for a complete meal. Prepare the chicken and let it stand, refrigerated, overnight, before stir-frying, and you'll have a really quick and tasty meal.

Good for: Constipation, menstrual problems

Healing Properties: Practitioners of Chinese medicine often prescribe walnuts to relieve constipation because the oils they contain lubricate the intestines. From a Western perspective, there's good news and bad news about walnuts: although they are rich in saturated fats, walnuts also contain about 5 percent alpha-linolenic acid, a source of omega-3 fatty acids. These acids are helpful in reducing the amount of "bad cholesterol" circulating in your blood.

PREPARATION: 15 minutes   STANDING TIME: 5 minutes
COOKING TIME: 8 minutes   SERVES: 4

12 ounces boneless, skinless chicken breast
2 teaspoons thin soy sauce
2 teaspoons dry sherry
2 teaspoons cornstarch
¼ teaspoon ground black pepper
2 tablespoons soybean oil
½ cup walnut halves
1 teaspoon minced ginger
1 scallion, green and white parts, minced
⅓ cup chicken broth or water

1. Cut the chicken into ½-inch cubes. In a small bowl, combine the chicken with the soy sauce, sherry, cornstarch, and pepper. Mix well and let stand 5 minutes.

2. Heat a wok until just smoking, add the oil, and stir-fry the walnuts, tossing frequently, about 30 seconds. Remove to paper towels and drain.

3. Return the wok to the heat, add the ginger and scallions, and stir-fry until aromatic, about 10 seconds. Add the chicken and cook, tossing frequently, until the chicken turns white and is cooked through, about 5 to 7 minutes.

4. Add the chicken broth, return to a boil, and cook 1 minute or until the sauce thickens. Add the walnuts, tossing to blend well. Serve.

— *Braised Duck with Cinnamon, Garlic, and Bamboo* —

To make this dish lower in fat, prepare the duck a day ahead and chill the dish overnight. This will allow any fat that remains to rise to the top so that you can remove it. Then you can reheat the dish on top of the stove or in the oven.

Good for: Colds and coughs, menopausal symptoms, chronic fatigue

Healing Properties: Cinnamon can help relieve cold and congestion by inducing perspiration and warming the upper region of the body. From a Western and Eastern perspective, the garlic, too, has medicinal qualities with respect to treating colds: it contains substances that boost the immune system as well as work as antibiotics. Bamboo shoots have a special benefit: their coolness helps to modify the warm or hot energy of the duck and, therefore, strikes a balance between the ingredients.

PREPARATION: 25 minutes   COOKING TIME: 1½ hours   SERVES: 4

---

1 duck, about 5 pounds
2 heads garlic
¼ cup dark soy sauce
½ cup rice wine
1 teaspoon ground black pepper
2 teaspoons fennel seeds
2 pieces dried tangerine peel
1 star anise
1 cinnamon stick
2 slices ginger
½ cup water
2 cups sliced bamboo shoots

1. Cut the duck into pieces, discarding the back bone and as much of the fat as possible. Leave the skin on.

2. Peel the garlic cloves and lightly crush.

3. Place the duck and garlic in a heavy casserole, add the soy sauce, and toss to coat the duck. Add the rice wine, pepper, fennel seeds, tangerine peel, star anise, cinnamon stick, ginger and the water. Stir to blend.

4. Preheat the oven to 350 degrees. Bring the casserole to a boil on top of the stove. Scatter the bamboo shoots over the duck, cover, and braise in the oven until the duck is tender when pricked with a fork, about 1 hour.

— Five-Spice Roast Duck —

This is a home recipe for the ducks you see hanging in the windows of Chinatown markets. Traditionally, roasts were never done at home as most kitchens did not have ovens. For a really crisp duck, follow the recipe with care and use a rack. About two cups of fat will be rendered. If you have a convection oven, use it, as this will result in the crispiest duck.

Good for: Indigestion, sinusitis

Healing Properties: Maltose, which is a sweetener made from barley or rice, is considered a warming, sweet food that has the potential to slow down the attack of acute symptoms and soothe the stomach and spleen. Five-spice powder consists of star anise, Chinese cinnamon, cloves, fennel, and Szechuan peppercorns. As you might suspect, these aromatic spices help relieve the stuffiness and pain associated with sinusitis.

PREPARATION: 10 minutes   STANDING TIME: 4 to 6 hours
COOKING TIME: 2 hours   SERVES: 4 to 6

1 cup maltose
1 whole duck, about 5 pounds
2 tablespoons soy sauce
1 tablespoon five-spice powder
1 teaspoon black pepper

1. In a large pot, bring 6 to 8 quarts of water to a boil. Add the maltose and stir to dissolve. Return the water to a boil and plunge the duck into it, making sure that the whole duck is submerged. Immediately remove the duck and pat dry with paper towels. The skin of the duck will have tightened.

2. In a small bowl, combine the soy sauce, five-spice powder, and pepper.

3. Place the duck on a rack over a roasting pan and paint its surface with the soy mixture. Let it air dry for 4 to 6 hours, brushing with the soy mixture periodically. The skin of the duck should feel like parchment.

4. Preheat the oven to 450 degrees. Roast the duck, breast side up, for 10 to 15 minutes or until light brown. Reduce the oven heat to 350 degrees and continue roasting the duck until the juices run clear when you prick the thigh, 1 to 1½ hours.

5. Remove the duck from the oven. Let stand 30 minutes before carving.

▣ Eggs

— Steamed Custard with Garlic Chives and Shrimp —

Smooth, creamy, and yet with a little spice and bite thanks to the chives and shrimp, this "comfort food" is sure to please your palate whether you suffer from digestive problems or not.

Good for: Anemia, diarrhea

Healing Properties: Eggs have an ascending nature, which means they influence energy and fluids to move higher in the body. Thus they are often used in Chinese medicine to cure diarrhea. In both Eastern and Western medicine, eggs are considered a good source of protein, which can help build the blood.

PREPARATION: 10 minutes   COOKING TIME: 15 minutes
SERVES: 2

¼ pound medium shrimp
4 eggs
2 tablespoons boiled water, cooled
2 teaspoons thin soy sauce
¼ teaspoon ground white pepper
¾ cup garlic chives, cut into ¼-inch pieces, about 3 ounces
1 teaspoon sesame oil

1. Peel and devein the shrimp; chop coarsely.
2. In a bowl, beat the eggs with the tepid water lightly with *one* chopstick. Do not let any foam form. Stir in the soy sauce and pepper. Stir in the shrimp and chives.
3. Lightly grease a heatproof shallow bowl with the sesame oil.
4. Pour the egg mixture into the greased bowl, place in a steam-

er basket, cover, and steam in a wok with just enough water to touch the bottom of the basket. Cook the custard 15 minutes. Keep the flame low, so the custard gently sets but does not become spongy. Serve.

— *Egg White Crab "Omelet" with Button Mushrooms and Bean Sprouts* —

This is really more of a flat omelet or frittata. If you use a nonstick skillet, the omelet will slide off the pan easily for an attractive presentation.

Good for: Diarrhea

Healing Properties: Chinese practitioners often prescribe a combination of eggs and mushrooms to treat diarrhea.

PREPARATION: 20 minutes   COOKING TIME: 8 minutes   SERVES: 4

---

1 10-ounce box of white button mushrooms
½ pound crabmeat
1 cup bean sprouts
2 tablespoons soybean oil
1 tablespoon minced shallots
1 teaspoon minced ginger
2 scallions, white and green parts, cut into 1-inch pieces
1 teaspoon salt
½ teaspoon pepper
8 egg whites
1 teaspoon black sesame seeds
4 sprigs fresh cilantro

1. Clean the mushrooms with a damp paper towel, remove the stems, and slice. Pick over the crabment to remove any bits of cartilage and shell. Rinse the bean sprouts and dry them in a salad spinner.

2. Preheat the broiler.

3. In a skillet, heat 1 tablespoon of the oil; add the shallots and ginger and sauté 30 seconds. Add the mushrooms and cook, stirring, until the mushrooms are soft and most of the liquid has evaporated. Add the crabmeat, scallions, bean sprouts, ½ teaspoon of the salt, and the pepper. Stir to mix well. Cook until heated through and the sprouts have wilted a little.

4. Beat the egg whites with the remaining salt until stiff but not dry.

5. In a clean, nonstick, 10-inch skillet, heat the remaining oil over medium heat. Spread half the egg whites to form a layer on the pan. Spread the crabmeat mixture evenly over the egg white layer and cover with the remaining egg whites. Sprinkle with black sesame seeds and run under the broiler to lightly brown the top. Slide the omelet onto a serving platter. Garnish with cilantro sprigs just before serving.

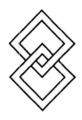

Resource Guide

In picking up this book and learning about Chinese medicine and cuisine, you've entered a whole new world—one you might need help getting around. This Resource Guide lists mail-order companies that offer cooking utensils and tools, as well as other books that will supplement your knowledge about Chinese culture and healing traditions.

• Equipment and Ingredients

If you have trouble finding the right cleaver, wok, or other cooking tools, or equipment or ingredients necessary to prepare the recipes in this book, contact one or more of the following companies and request a catalog.

California

Chong Kee Jan Company
838 Grant Avenue
San Francisco, CA 94108
(415) 982-1432

Wing Chong Lung Co. Grocery
922 South San Pedro Street
Los Angeles, CA 94108

The Wok Shop
718 Grant Avenue
San Francisco, CA 94108
(415) 989-3797

Connecticut

China Bowl Trading Co., Inc.
P.O. Box 454
Westport, CT 06881
(203) 222-0381

China Trading
271 Crown Street
New Haven, CT 06511
(203) 865-9465

Illinois

Oriental Food Market
7411 North Clark Street
Chicago, IL 60657
(312) 274-2826

Treasure Island
3460 North Broadway
Chicago, IL 60657
(312) 327-3880

Massachusetts

Joyce Chen, Unlimited
423 Great Road
Acton, MA 01720
(800) 828-0368
(508) 263-6922

Sun Sun Co. 18 Oxford Street
Boston, MA 02111
(617) 426-6494

Legal Sea Foods Market
5 Cambridge Center
Kendall Square
Cambridge, MA 02139
(617) 864-3400

New York

Kam Man Food Products
200 Canal Street
New York, NY 10013
(212) 571-0330

Katagiri and Co.
224 East 59th Street
New York, NY 10012
(212) 755-3566

Mon Fong Wo Company
36 Pell Street
New York, NY 10013
(212) 962-5418

• *Vitamins and Herbs*

Bio-San Laboratories
P.O. Box 325
Organic Park
Derry, NH 03038
(603) 432-5022

Mayway Trading Company
780 Broadway
San Francisco, CA 95073
(415) 788-3646

Dragon River Herbal
P.O. Box 74, Highway 285
Ojo Caliente, NM 87549
(505) 583-2118

McZand Herbal
P.O. Box 5312
Santa Monica, CA 90409
(800) 800-0405

K'an Herb Company
6001 Butler Lane
Scotts Valley, CA 95066
(408) 438-9450
Fax: (408) 438-9457

• *Organizations for Chinese Medicine*

American Academy of Medical Acupuncture
5820 Wilshire Boulevard, Suite 500
Los Angeles, CA 90036
(800) 521-AAMA

American Foundation of Traditional Chinese Medicine
505 Beach Street
San Francisco, CA 94133
(415) 776-0502

National Commission for the Certification of Acupuncturists
1424 16th Street NW
Washington, DC 20036
(202) 232-1404

National Oriental Medicine and Acupuncture Alliance
636 Prospect Avenue
Hartford, CT 06105
(203) 232-4825

Qigong Institute/East-West Academy of Healing Arts
450 Sutter Street
San Francisco, CA 94108
(415) 788-2227

• Further Reading

Beinfeld, Harriet, and Efrem Korngold. *Between Heaven and Earth: A Guide to Chinese Medicine.* New York: Ballantine Books, 1991.

Borysenko, Joan. *Minding the Body, Mending the Mind.* New York: Bantam Books, 1988.

Braverman, Eric R., M.D., and Carl C. Pfeiffer, M.D. *The Healing Nutrients Within.* New Canaan, Conn.: Keats Publishing, 1987.

Castleman, Michael. *The Healing Herbs.* Emmaus, Pa.: Rodale Press, 1991.

Cleary, Thomas. *I Ching: The Book of Change.* Boston: Shambhala, 1992.

————. *Vitality, Energy, Spirit.* Boston: Shambhala, 1992.

————. *Awakening to the Tao.* Boston: Shambhala, 1988.

Colbin, Annemarie. *Food and Healing.* New York: Ballantine, 1986.

Fratkin, Jake. *Chinese Classics: Popular Chinese Herbal Formulas.* Boulder, Colo.: Shya Publications, 1990.

Goldberg Group. *Alternative Medicine: The Definitive Guide.* Puyallap, Wash. Future Medicine Publishing, 1993.

Haas, Elson M., M.D. *Staying Healthy with Nutrition.* Berkeley, Calif.: Celestial Arts Publishing, 1992.

Hoffman, David. *The Herbal Handbook.* Rochester, Vt.: Healing Arts Press, 1987.

Kaptchuk, Ted. *The Web That Has No Weaver: Understanding Chinese Medicine.* New York: Congdon and Weed, 1992.

Lappe, Frances Moore. *Diet for a Small Planet.* New York: Ballantine, 1982.

McNamara, Sheila. *Traditional Chinese Medicine.* New York: Basic Books, 1996.

Monte, Tom, and editors of *EastWest Natural Health. World Medicine: The EastWest Guide to Healing Your Body.* New York: Tarcher/Perigee, 1993.

Moyers, Bill. *Healing and the Mind.* New York: Doubleday, 1993.

Pitchford, Paul. *Healing with Whole Foods: Oriental Traditions and Modern Nutrition.* Berkeley, Calif.: North Atlantic Books, 1993.

Reid, Daniel. *Chinese Herbal Medicine.* Boston: Shambhala Publications, 1986.

————. *The Complete Book of Chinese Health and Healing: Guarding the Three Treasures.* Boston: Shambhala Publications, 1994.

Ross, Rosa Lo San. *Beyond Bok Choy: A Cook's Guide to Asian Vegetables.* New York: Artisan, 1996.

Stanway, Penny, M.D. *Healing Foods for Common Ailments.* Toronto: Key Porter Books, 1995.

Tang, Stephen, and Richard Craze. *Chinese Herbal Medicine.* New York: Berkley, 1995.

Weil, Andrew. *Natural Health, Natural Medicine.* New York: Houghton-Mifflin, 1990.

Williams, Tom, Ph.D. *Chinese Medicine.* Rockport, Mass.: Element, 1995.

Yan-kit. *Classic Chinese Cookbook: A Complete Guide to the Equipment, Ingredients, Recipes, and Techniques.* New York: Dorling Kindersley, 1993.

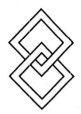 *Glossary*

Acupuncture: The treatment in Chinese medicine that frees up and influences the flow of qi by the insertion of fine needles into specific points in the body.

Allergy: A hypersensitive or exaggerated reaction to exposure to certain substances.

Anemia: A deficiency of hemoglobin, the number of red blood cells, or the amount of blood, leading to a lack of oxygen in the body cells.

Antibiotic: A drug used to treat bacterial infection.

Antibody: A protein produced by the body's immune system in response to an intruder or any cell that the body perceives as harmful; serves to protect the body from disease caused by viruses, bacteria, and other intruders.

Antihistamine: A drug that blocks the action of histamine, a chemical produced in large amounts during allergy attacks; used to treat allergies.

Antioxidants: Chemical compounds that prevent oxygen from reacting with other compounds. Some antioxidants have the potential to protect against cancer because they neutralize free radicals, chemicals that destroy or corrupt normal cells.

Arthritis: A term used in Western medicine to describe more than a hundred different conditions involving inflammation of the joints and, in some cases, other body tissues and systems as well.

Aspirin: A drug used in Western medicine to relieve pain and lower fever; an anti-inflammatory.

Autoimmune disease: A disorder in which the body produces antibodies against its own tissues.

Bacteria: One-celled microscopic organisms, some of which cause disease according to Western medical theory.

Beta-carotene: A nutrient that the body converts to vitamin A. It is found in orange and yellow fruits and vegetables such as cantaloupe, carrots, and green leafy vegetables.

Bile: The bitter fluid secreted by the liver to aid in digestion.

Biofeedback: A technique that uses feedback from specially designed equipment to detect physiological changes, such as raised blood pressure or pain response, in order to facilitate conscious control over these functions.

Bladder: The organ that contains the urine before it is excreted through the urethra.

Blood pressure: The force exerted by the blood against the arterial walls as it flows through the body.

Blood sugar level: The amount and concentration of glucose (sugar) in the blood.

Bronchitis: Inflammation of the air passages (bronchii) of the lungs.

Caffeine: A substance that stimulates the central nervous system and is present in coffee, tea, chocolate, and many soft drinks.

Candidiasis: A yeast infection caused by the *Candida* fungus. Also called **thrush.**

Canker sore: An ulcerlike sore on the mucous membrane of the mouth or lips.

Carbohydrates: Organic compounds that include starches, cellulose, and sugars. Sugars are called **simple carbohydrates** and are found in such foods as fruits and table sugar. **Complex carbohydrates** (starches) are composed of large numbers of sugar molecules and are found in grains, legumes, and vegetables like potatoes, squash, and corn.

Cardiovascular: Pertaining to the heart and blood vessels.

Cartilage: A resilient but firm connective or fibrous tissue that covers the ends of bones.

Channels: In traditional Chinese medicine, invisible pathways of energy both on the surface of and within the body.

Cholesterol: Fatty substances found in the body's tissues and blood. In foods, only animal products contain cholesterol. An excess of certain kinds of cholesterol in the bloodstream can contribute to heart disease.

Chronic condition: A disorder that is deep-seated, long-standing, and recurrent.

Cirrhosis: Chronic inflammation and hardening of an organ, usually the liver.

Cold: In traditional Chinese medicine, a quality characterized by aversion to cold, desire for heat, hypoactivity, lethargy, and weakness.

Colitis: Inflammation of the colon (large intestine), characterized by bowel spasms, diarrhea, and constipation.

Congenital: Present at birth.

Constipation: A condition of infrequent and difficult bowel movements.

Corticosteroids: Drugs used to reduce inflammation. Related to the natural hormones cortisone and hydrocortisone, these powerful drugs may have serious side effects.

Dampness: In traditional Chinese medicine, a quality characterized by heaviness, swelling, fluid accumulation, watery stools, and phlegm.

Degenerative condition: A disorder in which there is a gradual and often irreversible process of decay.

Dermatitis: Any inflammation of the skin; may be manifested as a rash, scaling, blistering, etc.

Detoxification: The process of removing toxins—harmful substances—from the body.

Diabetes: A condition characterized by the body's inability to produce enough of the hormone insulin (which metabolizes sugar) or to use insulin properly.

Diuretic: Any substance that increases fluid output through urination.

Edema: An abnormal accumulation of fluid in the body that can produce swelling or inflammation.

Eight Indicators: In traditional Chinese medicine, the organization of diagnostic information according to the principles of yin/yang, interior/exterior, hot/cold, excess/deficiency.

Endocrine: Relating to glands that produce hormones, including the adrenal, pituitary, and thyroid.

Endorphins: Chemical substances produced by the central nervous system that suppress pain.

Enzyme: A protein secreted by cells that acts as a stimulator to induce chemical changes in other substances, but remains unchanged by the process.

Essential oil: A pure, concentrated, aromatic essence extracted from plants; used in aromatherapy.

Estrogen: A primarily female sex hormone produced by the ovaries, adrenal glands, and placenta. It controls the development of secondary sex characteristics, menstruation, and pregnancy.

Exterior (body): Includes body hair, skin, muscles, and peripheral blood vessels and nerves.

Fats: The body's most concentrated source of energy. All fats are made up of carbon, hydrogen, and oxygen atoms arranged in combinations of glycerol and fatty acids. Also known as **lipids.**

Fever: Abnormally high temperature, generally above 98.6° F or 37° C.

Fiber: The indigestible part of plants.

Five Elements: The five stages of life and nature corresponding to Water, Fire, Wood, Metal, and Earth, the seasons, climates, colors, organs, and emotions.

Flatulence: An overabundance of gas in the stomach or intestines.

Folic acid: A B-complex vitamin found in liver, kidney, green vegetables, and yeast.

Free radicals: Unstable molecules created by normal chemical processes in the body as well as by radiation and other environmental influences. The interaction of free radicals with DNA leads to impaired functioning or destruction of cells.

Fungus: A form of vegetable life that can be both healthful and disease producing.

Gastric: Pertaining to the stomach.

Gastric acid: Secretion of the stomach containing enzymes and acid to aid in digestion.

Gastritis: Inflammation of the stomach.

Genetic: Hereditary; pertaining to the passage of traits through successive generations.

Gout: A metabolic disorder related to arthritis in which an overabundance of uric acid in the blood leads to the deposit of urate crystals in the joints.

Halitosis: Technical term for bad breath.

Harmony: The existence of balance and creativity in nature and in the human body.

Hay fever: An allergic reaction to pollens in which the mucous membranes of the eyes, nose, and throat become inflamed.

Heat: In traditional Chinese medicine, a quality characterized by aversion to heat, desire for cold, hyperactivity, dehydration, constipation, insomnia, and restlessness.

Hemoglobin: The oxygen-carrying protein of the blood found in red blood cells.

Hepatitis: An inflammatory disease of the liver.

Herpes simplex: Recurring infection caused by herpes virus. Type I involves blisterlike sores, usually around the mouth, called cold sores. Type II involves the mucous membranes of the genitalia and can be spread by sexual contact.

Hormone: A chemical produced by a gland. Each type stimulates a target organ or organs to a specific action.

Immune system: The body's line of defense against disease comprised of several different blood cells as well as antibodies.

Indigestion: An abnormality in the digestive process causing gas, feelings of heaviness, and sometimes nausea.

Inflammation: Redness and swelling of a part of the body resulting from injury or disease.

Insomnia: Difficulty in falling or staying asleep.

Insulin: A hormone secreted by the pancreas in response to elevated blood sugar levels.

Interior (body): Includes bones, visceral organs, glands, major blood vessels and nerves, and body cavities.

Irritable bowel syndrome: A condition that occurs when the regular rhythmic contractions that normally propel waste through the intestines become irregular, resulting in constipation or diarrhea and other abdominal disorders.

Ke Cycle: In traditional Chinese medicine, the interaction of the Five Elements whereby one element controls, inhibits, and regulates another.

Menopause: The state resulting in the cessation of menstruation and ovulation, and the marked decline in the production of the hormone estrogen.

Moxa: Dried leaves of mugwort, an herb used in traditional Chinese acupuncture; moxa is heated, then held near an acupuncture point to warm and tonify energy, a process called **moxibustion.**

Nausea: A feeling of sickness in the stomach.

Nutrients: Components necessary for all bodily functions that must be obtained from foods or supplements since the body cannot manufacture them.

Omega-3 fatty acids: A unique group of fatty acids found in fish oil and some seeds. Omega-3's in fish oil significantly reduce hardening of the arteries (atherosclerosis) by making blood components called platelets less likely to stick to blood vessels.

Palpation: Physical examination using the hands or feet to feel for tissue abnormalities.

Pathogen: A disease-causing agent.

Pattern of Disharmony: In traditional Chinese medicine, the diagnosis of disease based on the categories of yin/yang, Five Elements, Seven Emotions, and Eight Indicators.

Proteins: Compounds present in the body and in foods that are complex combinations of amino acids. Protein is essential for life. Foods that supply the body with protein include animal products, grains, legumes, and vegetables.

Qi: In traditional Chinese medicine, the life-force or energy of the body, which circulates through the body's channels.

Sheng Cycle: In traditional Chinese medicine, the Five Element interaction whereby one element produces, gives rise to, or nourishes another.

Tao: A philosophical term that denotes the universe as an undifferentiated whole.

Tissue: A collection of cells designed to perform one specific function.

Toxin: Any substance that is harmful or poisonous to the body; often used to describe waste materials in the bloodstream which, when accumulated, can cause health problems.

Vitamins: Organic substances that the body requires to regulate metabolic functions.

Wind: In traditional Chinese medicine, a quality characterized by aversion to drafts, spasms, migratory pains, dizziness, headache, flu symptoms, and numbness.

Yang: One of the two fundamental, polar forces that organize the universe. Yang qualities include heat, dryness, activity, growth, expansion, and fullness.

Yang organs: In Chinese medicine, the small intestine, gallbladder, stomach, large intestine, and urinary bladder.

Yin: One of the two fundamental, polar forces that organize the universe. Yin qualities include coldness, fluid, and inertia.

Yin organs: In Chinese medicine, the liver, heart, spleen, lungs, and kidneys.

Yin/yang: Mutually interdependent forces; the principle of duality that organizes the universe and the process that characterizes life.

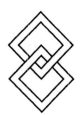

Index

A

acetylcysteine, 76
acupoints, 25
acupressure massage, 26, 72-73, 105
acupuncture
  for anemia, 66
  for cold sores, 83
  for flu, 101
  for hay fever, 103
  for headache, 105
  for hemorrhoids, 107
  for herpes, 112
  for indigestion, 117
  introduction to U.S., 7-8
  for menstrual problems, 124
  for pain (chronic), 129
  for psoriasis, 131
  technique, 25-26
acyclovir, 111
akebia, 133
alcoholism, and folic-acid deficiency, 65
allergies
  causes of, 35
  food, 78, 92, 104, 115
  hay fever, 102-03, 104
  sinus infection, 132
Aloe vera, 95, 105, 131
American Dietetic Association, 41
amino acid, 37
analgesics, 128
anemia, 64-67
  Chinese medicine, 66-67
  healing recipes, 67, 145, 147, 149, 158, 161, 181, 185, 211
  Western medicine, 64-66

Angelica
  pubescens, 66, 73, 95, 105-06, 133
  sinensis, 121-22, 124
anger, cause of disease, 19-20
anise, star, 55
antacids, 98, 116
antibiotics, 76, 78, 92, 94, 96, 98, 105, 134, 208
antihistamines, 102, 105
anti-inflammatory drugs, 69, 71-72
  healing recipes, 171
  herbal, 27
antioxidants, 43, 85, 100, 133, 158, 159
anxiety, 20, 116, 118
apricot, 38
arthritis, 67-71
  causes of, 18, 35, 43
  Chinese medicine, 70-71
  healing recipes, 71, 182, 193
  pain, 122, 123
  Western medicine, 67-70
Asarum sieboldii, 66, 85, 97
asparagus, healing properties of, 38
aspirin, 72, 76, 82, 84, 128
astragalus, 81, 91

B

back pain, 122
  Chinese medicine, 72-73
  healing recipes, 73
  Western medicine, 64-66
  See also pain, chronic
bad breath, 73-75, 86
  Chinese medicine, 74-75
  healing recipes, 75, 166

bad breath *(continued)*
Western medicine, 74
bai he wan (Preserver Harmony Pill),
126
bai ji (Bletilla striata), 112, 131
bai shao (white peony), 122
ba jeng san (Eight Orthodox Powder),
135
balance
of Five Elements, 16
nutritional, 30-34
yin-yang, 10-12
balloon flower, 77
bamboo shoots
in Chinese cooking, 55
*duck, braised with cinnamon, garlic
and, 208-09*
bamboo steamer, 58
banana, 38, 79
basil
*coconut soup with peppermint
sprigs, 143-44*
healing properties of, 70, 143
bean curd
cubes, with chicken sauce, 155-56
*dried sticks, with Buddha's Delight,
160-61*
*dried sticks, and ginkgo nut congee,
174-75*
fresh, 51
healing properties of, 119, 155,
174, 198
*hot and sour soup, vegetarian, 148-
49*
oyster, and mushroom stew, 196-97
puffed, 51
and spinach soup, 149-50
bean paste
hot, with eggplant, 162-63
red, 51
beans
black, fermented, 51
and flatulence, 98, 99
healing properties of, 37
long, with scallops, 198-99
See also black bean sauce
bean sprouts
egg white crab "omelet" with button

mushrooms and, 212-13
healing properties of, 178, 182
*mung, brown rice with cabbage
ribbons and, 178-79*
soybean sprouts with beef, 182-83
bedwetting, 21
beef
healing properties of, 39, 66, 181
*hoisin, with red and green peppers,
181-82*
soup, essence, 145
with soybean sprouts, 182-83
bee pollen, 103
beet, 38
Beinfeld, Harriet, 8
beta-carotene, 43, 168, 171
Between Heaven and Earth (Beinfeld
and Korngold), 8
beverages, 49, 92, 134
See also fluid intake; tea
bioflavonoids, 103, 162
bitter foods, 34, 156
black bean sauce
with braised pork, 186
clams and mussels in, 189-90
bladder
emotional causes of disease, 20-21
in Five Elements system, 15, 16, 72
and nutrition, 37
urinary tract infection, 134-35
Bletilla striata, 112, 131
bloating, 91, 97, 98, 123, 124, 195
blood circulation, 143
blood loss, and iron deficiency, 64
blood pressure, 113
bo he (mint), 97, 101, 133
bok choy
in Chinese cooking, 56
with garlic, 158-59
bran, 87
breath fresheners, natural, 74, 75
broccoli
Chinese, 55-56
healing properties of, 38, 43, 159
with sesame dressing, 159-60
bronchitis, 75-77
Chinese medicine, 77
healing recipes, 77, 155, 177, 199

Western medicine, 75-77
Buddha's Delight with dried bean curd sticks, 160-61

C

cabbage
Chinese, 56
Chinese, bok choy with garlic, 158-59
flowering white, and Chinese celery, with cellophane noodles, 171-72
healing properties of, 38, 43, 178
ribbons, brown rice with mung bean sprouts and, 178-79
caffeine, 66, 70, 105, 124
calcium, 69, 72, 133, 149
calories, 46
cancer, and nutrition, 42, 43
Candida albicans, 78, 97
candidiasis (yeast overgrowth), 77-80
Chinese medicine, 79
and flatulence, 98
healing recipes, 79-80, 156, 178, 198, 200
Western medicine, 78-79
carp, steamed, on mustard greens, 188-89
catnip, Japanese, 106
cauliflower, 43
celery
Chinese, and flowering white cabbage, with cellophane noodles, 171-72
healing properties of, 38
cellophane noodles with Chinese celery and flowering white cabbage, 171-72
chai hu (hare's ear), 101, 122
chamomile tea, 92
che chien dze (plantain), 77
chicken
broth, white fungus in, 152-53
"cake," steamed, 202-03
cubes with lichee and plum sauce, 203-04
healing properties of, 39, 76, 133, 202, 203

legs with pineapple and mandarin peel, 205-06
sauce, with bean curd cubes, 155-56
soup, ginseng, 147
soup, soba noodles with mustard greens, 177-78
with walnuts, 206-07
chien tsao (Indian madder), 110
chili paste
in Chinese cooking, 51-52
healing properties of, 155
chili powder, 54
Chinese cooking
ingredients in, 50-58
mail-order sources for, 215-17
serving style in, 48-49
steaming, 58
stir-frying, 58-59
tools for, 49-50
Chinese medicine
acupuncture/acupressure therapy, 7-8, 25-26, 72-73
and anemia, 66-67
and arthritis, 70
and back pain, 72-73
and bad breath, 74-75
and bronchitis, 77
and candidiasis, 79
causes of disease, 17-21
and chronic fatigue syndrome, 81-82
and cold sores, 83
and common cold, 85-86
and constipation, 87-88
and diabetes, 90-91
diagnosis in, 21-25
and diarrhea, 92-93
and dizziness, 95
and ear infections, 96-97
and Five Elements system, 13-16
and flatulence, 98-99
and flu, 100-01
goal of treatment, 12
and hay fever, 103
and headache, 105-06
and hemorrhoids, 107-08
and hepatitis, 109-10
and herpes simplex type 2, 112
holistic approach of, 8, 9

Chinese medicine *(continued)*
and hypertension, 114-15
and indigestion, 117
information sources on, 218-20
and insomnia, 119
life force (qi) in, 12-13, 16
and menopausal symptoms, 121-22
and menstrual problems, 125
and natural law, 10
and nausea, 126
organizations for, 217-18
and pain (chronic), 129
and psoriasis, 131
qi-gong therapy, 28
and sinus infection, 133
and urinary tract infection, 135
vs Western medicine, 8-9
yin/yang balance in, 10-12
See also herbal remedies; nutrition
and diet, Eastern
Chinese yam, 112
chives
Chinese, 56
garlic, flowers, with pork liver, 185
chlorophyll, 158
cholesterol, 42, 43-45
chopping board, 49
chopsticks, eating with, 48-49
chronic fatigue syndrome (CFS), 78,
80- 82
Chinese medicine, 81-82
healing recipes, 82, 145, 187, 208
Western medicine, 80-81
cilantro
as breath freshener, 75, 166
forms of, 54
healing properties of, 117, 166
and slivered radish salad, 166
cinnamon
*duck, braised with garlic, bamboo
and, 208-09*
healing properties of, 70-71, 85,
208
circulation, and Five Elements system,
15

clams
healing properties of, 39, 189, 195
*and mussels in black bean sauce,
189-90*
cleaver, 49
coconut
milk, 143, 179
rice, sweet, 179-80
*soup, basil, with peppermint sprigs,
143-44*
Codonopsis dangshen, 115
cold, common, 18, 75, 84-86, 132
Chinese medicine, 85-86
healing recipes, 86, 142, 151, 152,
165, 167, 175, 177, 192, 200,
208
Western medicine, 84-85
cold sores, 82-84
Chinese medicine, 83
healing recipes, 84, 162, 190, 202,
203
Western medicine, 82-83
cold (yin), 18, 24
colitis, 20
colon cancer, 42
congee
basic, 173-74
ginkgo nut and bean curd stick, 174-75
for nausea, 126
constipation, 78, 86-88, 108, 122
causes of, 20, 35, 86, 106
Chinese medicine, 87-88, 124
chronic, 86
healing recipes, 88, 149, 151, 152,
159, 171, 178, 206
Western medicine, 87
cooking. *See* Chinese cooking
copper, 66, 69
coriander. *See* cilantro
cornstarch, 53
corticosteroids, 102
cough
bronchitis, 75
common cold, 84-86
flu, 99
hay fever, 102
healing recipes, 142, 151, 152, 165,
167, 171, 188, 208

crab "omelet," egg white, with button
mushrooms and bean sprouts, 212-
13
cramps, 18, 78, 97, 195
cranberry juice, 134
cysteine, 76
cystitis, 134

D

da dzao (Chinese jujube), 115
da huang (rhubarb root), 83
dairy products, 85, 87, 132
and cholesterol, 44
in Eastern diet, 38-39
dampness conditions, 18, 35, 79, 81,
83, 93, 109, 112
dang gui (Angelica sinensis), 121-22,
124
dang sheng (Codonopsis dangshen),
115
da suan (garlic), 85
dates
Buddha's Delight with dried bean
curd sticks, 160-61
healing properties of, 67, 161
dehydration, 18, 92
diabetes, 42, 78, 88-91, 118
Chinese medicine, 90-91
healing recipes, 91, 143, 164, 165,
185, 187, 196, 197, 202, 203
health problems related to, 88
Western medicine, 89-90
diarrhea, 18, 34, 37, 39, 78, 91-93,
95, 108
Chinese medicine, 92-93
healing recipes, 93, 141, 147, 158,
173, 174, 175, 211, 212
symptoms of, 91
Western medicine, 92
diet. See nutrition and diet, Eastern;
nutrition and diet, Western
di fu dze (Belvedere cypress), 135
digestion
and bad breath, 74
fiber in, 42
and Five Elements system, 14, 15
and flatulence, 97, 205

of legumes, 37
pungent foods in, 33
See also diarrhea; indigestion
disease
emotional causes of (Seven
Emotions), 19-21
environmental causes of (Six Evils),
17-19, 85
diuretics, 123, 165, 182
dizziness
causes of, 20, 94, 95, 112
Chinese medicine, 95, 122
healing recipes, 95, 171
Western medicine, 94-95
drug treatment
of arthritis, 69
of back pain, 72-73
of bronchitis, 76
of cold sores, 82-83
of diabetes, 89, 90
of hay fever, 102
of herpes, 111
of hypertension, 113
of insomnia, 118
of menstrual problems, 123
pain (chronic), 128
of yeast infection, 78
dryness (yang), 18
duck
braised, with cinnamon, garlic, and
bamboo, 208-09
five-spice roast, 209-10
healing properties of, 39
du huo (Angelica pubescens), 66, 73,
95, 105-06, 133
du jung (eucommia), 73
dzang hung hua (Tibetan saffron), 122

E

ear infections, 94, 95-97
Chinese medicine, 96-97
healing recipes, 97
Western medicine, 96
Earth element, 14-15, 16
Eastern medicine. See Chinese medicine
edema, healing recipes for, 179, 189

egg(s)
  and cholesterol, 44-45
  custard, oysters steamed in, 197-98
  *custard, steamed, with garlic
    chives and shrimp, 211-12*
  healing properties of, 39, 66, 93,
    117, 119, 197, 211
  *white "omelet," crab, with button
    mushrooms and bean sprouts,
    212-13*
eggplant
  healing properties of, 38, 108, 162
  with hot bean paste, 162-63
Eight Indicators, 23-25
Elsholtzia splendens, 101
emotional conditions, and disease, 19-
  21
emphysema, 76
environmental conditions, and disease,
  17-19, 85
Ephedra sinica, 103
Epstein-Barr virus, 80
estrogen replacement therapy (ERT),
  120-21
exercise
  acupressure, 72-73
  for constipation, 87, 88
  for diabetes, 89, 90
  for hemorrhoids, 107
  for hypertension, 115
  for menopausal symptoms, 121
  for pain (chronic), 128
  relaxation, 105, 115
extracts, herbal, 27

          F
fat, dietary
  in Chinese diet, 39-40
  and cholesterol, 44-45
  for constipation, 87
  daily intake, 46
  types of, 40, 45-46
fatigue. *See* chronic fatigue syndrome
  (CFS)
fatty acids, 40, 45, 46, 91, 114, 146,
  206
fear, cause of disease, 20-21
fennel

healing properties of, 71, 193
  *seeds, fish, poached, with red wine
    sauce, 193-94*
fiber, dietary, 42, 98, 107
fire
  cause of disharmony, 19
  element, 14, 16
fish
  *carp, steamed, on mustard greens,
    188-89*
  and fat intake, 45-46
  healing properties of, 39, 114, 146
  with lemon sauce, 192-93
  oil, 46, 105
  poached, with red wine sauce, 193-94
  sauce, 57
  soup, fishball, 146-47
  wontons, -filled, 190-91
  See also seafood
Five Elements system, 13-16, 27
five-spice
  in Chinese cooking, 54
  duck, roast, 209-10
  healing properties of, 187, 209
  pork with Nam Yue, 187
flatulence, 97-99
  Chinese medicine, 98-99
  healing recipes, 99, 205
  Western medicine, 97-98
flavor of foods, 32-34
flaxseed oil, 91, 112
flu, 18, 75, 99-102
  Chinese medicine, 100-01
  healing recipes, 101-02, 142, 155,
    177, 188, 199, 200
  Western medicine, 100
fluid intake, 35, 41, 87, 92, 134
folic acid deficiency, 65
food allergy, 78, 92, 104, 115
Food Pyramid, 41, 46
free radicals, 43
fright, cause of disharmony, 21
fruit
  for bad breath, 75
  healing properties of, 37-38, 43,
    103, 192
  kumquats in perfumed syrup, 169-70
fungus

as diuretic, 26
healing properties of, 152
white, in chicken broth, 152-53

G
gallbladder, 37, 105, 109-10
in Five Elements system, 15, 16
gan jiang (dried ginger), 101
gan tsao (licorice), 77, 124
garlic
bok choy with, 158-59
*chive flowers, with pork liver, 185-
86*
*duck, braised with cinnamon, bam-
boo and, 208-09*
healing properties of, 38, 54, 67,
79, 85, 87, 93, 100, 158, 208
*squid with thin wheat noodles in
spicy sauce, 200-01*
gas, intestinal. *See* flatulence
Gastrodia and Uncaria Beverage, 115
geh gen tang (Pueraria Decoction), 85,
101
genistein, 43
genital herpes. *See* herpes simplex
type 2
gentian, 91
ginger(ed)
healing properties of, 54, 71, 85,
101, 105, 126, 142, 151, 165,
199, 200
honey, pumpkin, steamed, with, 165
root, 54
soup, and tomato, cold, 151-52
tea, 142
ginkgo nut(s), 56
and bean curd stick congee, 174-75
ginseng
chicken soup, 147
healing properties of, 67, 81, 91,
147
glucose tolerance test, 94
glutathione peroxidase, 43
gou jidze (Chinese wolfberry), 79
gout, 68-69, 70
governing vessel, 72
grains, healing properties of, 35-36,
87

grains of paradise, 117
grief, cause of disease, 20
gui pi wan (Returned Spleen Tablets),
66
Gynura pinnatifida, 110

H
halitosis. *See* bad breath
hare's ear, 101, 122
hay fever, 102-03
Chinese medicine, 103
healing recipes, 103, 143, 155
Western medicine, 102-03
headache, 104-06, 122, 128
causes of, 18, 20, 86, 104
Chinese medicine, 105-06, 122
healing recipes, 106, 146
Western medicine, 104-05
heart
causes of disease, 19, 20, 66, 118,
119
in Five Elements system, 14
and meat products, 39
heartburn, 78
heart disease, 42, 43, 88, 174
heat (yang), 18, 24
hemorrhoidectomy, 107
hemorrhoids, 34, 86, 106-08
Chinese medicine, 107-08
healing recipes, 108, 162, 189
Western medicine, 106-07
hepatitis, 108-10
Chinese medicine, 109-10
healing recipes, 110, 156, 186
Western medicine, 108-09
herbal remedies
for anemia, 66
for arthritis, 70
for back pain, 73
for bad breath, 75
for bronchitis, 77
for candidiasis, 79
in Chinese medicine, 26-27
for chronic fatigue syndrome, 81
for cold sores, 83
for common cold, 85
for diabetes, 91
for dizziness, 95

herbal remedies *(continued)*
for ear infections, 97
for flatulence, 99
for flu, 101
forms of, 27-28
for hay fever, 103
for headache, 105-06
for hepatitis, 110
for herpes, 112
for hypertension, 115
for indigestion, 117
for insomnia, 118-19
mail-order sources for, 217
for menopausal symptoms, 121-22
for menstrual problems, 124
for nausea, 126
for psoriasis, 131
for urinary tract infection, 135
See also specific herbs
herbs
in Chinese cooking, 53-55
mail-order sources for, 217
herpes simplex type 1, 82
herpes simplex type 2 (genital herpes),
110-12
and Chinese medicine, 112
healing recipes, 112, 141
Western medicine, 111
high blood pressure. *See* hypertension
high-density lipoprotein (HDL), 44,
45, 54
hoisin
beef with red and green peppers,
181-82
sauce, 57
holistic medicine, 8, 9
ho shou wu (Chinese cornbind), 73
hot and sour soup, vegetarian, 148-49
hsiang ru (Elsholtzia splendens), 101
hsi hsin (Asarum sieboldii), 66, 85, 97
hsuan fu hua (yellow starwort), 77
huang bai (philodendron bark), 83
huang chi (astragalus), 81, 91
huang jing (Polygonatum
cirrhifolium), 70
huang lien (mishmi bitter), 75
hu jiao (black pepper), 117
hypertension, 94, 104, 112-15

causes of, 20, 113, 114
Chinese medicine, 114-15
healing recipes, 115, 171, 174, 192
symptoms of, 105, 112
Western medicine, 113-14
hypoglycemia, 94, 164

I
indigestion, 115-18
causes of, 20, 31, 86, 115, 116, 117
Chinese medicine, 31, 117
healing recipes, 117-18, 142, 143,
147, 150, 164, 166, 169, 190,
192, 197, 209
Western medicine, 116-17
See also digestion
inflammatory bowel disease, 65
insomnia
causes of, 19, 86, 118, 119
Chinese medicine, 119, 122
healing recipes, 119, 148, 161, 196,
197
Western medicine, 118-19
insulin, 89, 90
interferon, 175
intestines
emotional causes of disease, 20
in Five Elements system, 14, 15, 72
iron, 69, 100, 181
absorption, 66
deficiency, 64-65, 66
Irritable bowel syndrome, 97, 98

J
jaundice, 108, 110
jian pi wan (Strengthen the Spleen
Pill), 126
jia wei shiao yao tang (Enhanced
Eliminate and Relax Decoction),
122
jie geng (balloon flower), 77
jih shih (trifoliate orange), 99
jing jie (Japanese catnip), 106
joy, cause of disease, 19

K
kale, 38, 43
Chinese, 55-56

Ke Cycle, 16
kidneys
  and diabetes, 88
  and ear infections, 96, 97
  emotional causes of disease, 20-21,
    66
  in Five Elements system, 15, 72
  and hypertension, 114
  and nutrition, 37, 135, 183
kohlrabi with swiss chard ribbons, 164
Korngold, Efrem, 8
kumquats
  healing properties of, 38, 169
  in perfumed syrup, 169-70

        L
lamb
  healing properties of, 135, 183
  *spicy, with wide rice noodles, 183-
    84*
laxatives, 87, 107
legumes, healing properties of, 36-37
lemon
  healing properties of, 38, 98, 192
  sauce, fish with, 192-93
leonurus (Siberian motherwort), 124
lettuce, 38
*lichee, chicken cubes with plum sauce
    and, 203-04*
licorice, 77, 85, 124
lily buds
  in Chinese cooking, 53
  *hot and sour soup, vegetarian, 148-
    49*
  for insomnia, 148
lime, 38
lipoprotein, 44, 45, 54
liver
  and anemia, 66
  causes of disease, 18, 19-20
  cholesterol production in, 44
  and constipation, 87
  and dizziness, 95
  in Five Elements system, 15-16
  and flatulence, 98-99
  and headache, 105, 106
  and hepatitis, 108-10
  and hypertension, 114

  and nausea, 126
  and nutrition, 37, 39, 186, 203
liver (food)
  healing properties of, 66, 185
  pork, with garlic chive flowers, 185
  lo mein with mushrooms, 175-76
low-density lipoprotein (LDL), 44, 45,
    54
lu hui (Aloe vera), 95, 105, 131
lung cancer, 43
lung dan tsao (gentian), 91
lungs
  causes of disease, 18, 19, 20, 133
  in Five Elements system, 15
  and nutrition, 33, 39
lysine, 83, 111

        M
magnesium, 72, 81
ma huang (Ephedra sinica), 103
maltose, 209
manganese, 69
massage, 26, 128
meadowsweet, 27
meat
  in Chinese diet, 38-39
  and cholesterol, 44
  healing properties of, 39
  healing recipes, 181-87
  See also beef; lamb; pork
meditation, 119, 124
melon
  bitter, steamed stuffed, 79, 156-57
  healing properties of, 153, 156
  winter, in Chinese cooking, 57
  winter, soup, 153-54
Meniere's disease, 94
menopausal symptoms, 120-22
  Chinese medicine, 121-22
  healing recipes, 122, 174, 208
  Western medicine, 120-21
menstrual problems, 122-25
  Chinese medicine, 125
  healing recipes, 126, 195, 203, 206
  symptoms of, 122
  Western medicine, 123-24
meridians, 12, 72
Metal Element, 15, 16

migraines, 104, 118
milk, 39, 85
minerals
    deficiency, 64-65
    essential, 42-43
mint
    healing properties of, 97, 101, 133
    See also peppermint; spearmint
monosaturated fats, 45
motion sickness, 169
moxibustion, 26
mu dan pi (tree peony), 103
mung bean sprouts, brown rice with cabbage ribbons and, 178-79
mushroom(s)
    button, egg white crab "omelet" with bean sprouts and, 212-13
    dried, 53
    healing properties of, 38, 93, 175, 196
    with lo mein, 175-76
    oyster, and bean curd stew, 196-97
    soup, hot and sour, vegetarian, 148-49
mussels
    and clams in black bean sauce, 189-90
    healing properties of, 189
    steamed in rice wine, 195
mustard greens
    carp, steamed, on, 188-89
    healing properties of, 177
    with soba noodles, 177-78
mu tong (akebia), 133

N

nam yue
    pork, five-spice, with, 187
    yam/taro root braised with, 168
nausea, 95, 99, 104, 108, 125-26
    Chinese medicine, 126
    healing recipes, 126, 147, 169, 173, 183
    Western medicine, 125-26
nicotine, and arthritis, 69-70
Nixon, Richard, in China, 7
nonsteroidal anti-inflammatory drugs
    (NSAIDs), 69, 71-72

noodles
    cellophane, with Chinese celery and flowering white cabbage, 171-72
    egg, 52-53
    lo mein with mushrooms, 175-76
    rice, 53
    rice, wide, with spicy lamb, 183-84
    soba, with mustard greens, 177-78
    thin wheat, with squid, in spicy sauce, 200-01
nori. *See* seaweed
nutmeg, 99, 117
nutrition and diet, Eastern, 28, 29, 30-40
    for anemia, 66-67
    for arthritis, 70-71
    for back pain, 73
    for bad breath, 75
    for bronchitis, 77
    for candidiasis, 79
    for chronic fatigue syndrome, 81-82
    for cold sores, 83
    for common cold, 85-86
    for constipation, 88
    for diabetes, 91
    for diarrhea, 93
    for ear infections, 97
    for flatulence, 99
    and flavor, 32-34
    fruits in, 37-38
    grains in, 35-36
    for hemorrhoids, 108
    for herpes, 112
    for hypertension, 115
    for indigestion, 117
    legumes in, 36-37
    meat/dairy in, 38-39
    for menopausal symptoms, 122
    for nausea, 126
    for pain (chronic), 129
    for psoriasis, 131
    for sinus infection, 133
    for urinary tract infection, 135
    vegetables in, 38
    and water intake, 35
    and yin/yang balance, 32, 34
nutrition and diet, Western, 30, 40-46

for anemia, 65-66
for arthritis, 69-70
for back pain, 72
for bad breath, 74
for bronchitis, 76-77
and cholesterol, 43-45
for cold sores, 83
for common cold, 85
for constipation, 87
for diabetes, 90
for diarrhea, 92
for dizziness, 94-95
for ear infections, 96
essential nutrients in, 41-42
fats in, 45-46
fiber in, 42
for flatulence, 98
for flu, 100
for hemorrhoids, 107
for herpes, 111
for hypertension, 114
for indigestion, 116-17
for menstrual problems, 123-24
for nausea, 126
for pain (chronic), 128-29
for psoriasis, 130-31
for sinus infection, 132-33
for urinary tract infection, 134
vitamins/minerais/phytochemicals
    in, 42-43, 65-66
for yeast infection, 78-79
nuts
ginkgo, 56
ginkgo, and bean curd stick congee,
    174-75
walnuts, chicken with, 206-07

O

oils, 40, 45-46, 57-58, 91, 114, 159
ointments, herbal, 28
olive oil, 45, 114
omega-3 fatty acids, 46, 91, 114, 206
oral contraceptives, 123
orange, 38
osteoarthritis, 67-68, 70
otitis media. *See* ear infections
oxygen, 41, 44

oyster(s)
healing properties of, 117, 119,
    196, 197
mushroom, and bean curd stew,
    196-97
steamed in egg custard, 197-98
oyster sauce, 57

P

pain, chronic, 127-29
Chinese medicine, 129
healing recipes, 129, 143, 167, 168,
    203
Western medicine, 127-29
See also back pain
palpitation, in physical exam, 23
papaya, 117
Parkinson's disease, 18
parsley
as breath freshener, 75
healing properties of, 97
peanut oil, 40, 45, 57-58
pensiveness, cause of disease, 20
peony
tree, 103
white, 122
peppermint
healing properties of, 97
sprigs, basil coconut soup with,
    143-44
peppers
healing properties of, 67, 135, 181
red and green, with hoisin beef,
    181-82
perspiration, and nutrition, 34
phenethyl isothiocyanate (PEITC), 43
philodendron bark, 83
physical examination, 21-25
phytochemicals, 43
pineapple
chicken legs with mandarin peel and,
    205-06
healing properties of, 38, 205
plantain, 77
plum(s)
healing properties of, 83, 110, 203
sauce, chicken cubes with lichee
    and, 203-04

polyunsaturated fats, 45-46
pork
    braised, with black bean sauce, 186
    five-spice, with nam yue, 187
    healing properties of, 110, 186
    liver with garlic chive flowers, 185
potato, 38
poultices, herbal, 28
pregnancy
    hemorrhoids in, 106
    iron deficiency in, 64
    nausea in, 125
prostaglandins, 128
prostate cancer, 43
protein, 72, 81-82, 96
    food sources of, 39, 108, 146, 174,
        175, 199, 211
psoriasis, 130-31
    Chinese medicine, 131
    healing recipes, 131, 159
    Western medicine, 130-31
pulse taking, 23
*pumpkin, steamed, with gingered
    honey, 165*
pungent foods, 33

Q
qi (life force), 12-13, 16, 25
qi-gong therapy, 28

R
radish
    healing properties of, 117, 166
    slivered, and cilantro salad, 166
raspberry, 38
relaxation exercises, 105, 115
ren shen. See ginseng
Reston, James, 7-8
rheumatism, 67-71
rheumatoid arthritis, 68, 70
rhubarb root, 83
rice
    *brown, with mung bean sprouts and
        cabbage ribbons, 178-79*
    in Chinese meal, 48
    coconut, sweet, 179-80
    healing properties of, 93, 135

long-grain, 52
    soup. *See* congee
    sticky (white glutinous), 52
*rice noodles, wide, with spicy lamb,
    183-84*
rou dou kou (nutmeg), 99, 117

S
saffron, Tibetan, 122
*salad, radish, slivered, and cilantro,
    166*
salicylates, 27
salt, 114, 123
salty foods, 34
san chi (Gynura pinnatifida), 110
sandalwood, 79
saturated fats, 44, 45, 206
sauces
    in Chinese cooking, 57-58
    lemon, with fish, 192-93
    *lichee and plum, with chicken cubes,
        203-04*
    red wine, fish poached with, 193-94
    See also black bean sauce
scallions, 55
scallops, with long beans, 198-99
seafood
    *crab "omelet," egg white, with
        button mushrooms and bean
        sprouts, 212-13*
    healing properties of, 39, 189, 196
    scallops with long beans, 198-99
    *squid with thin wheat noodles in
        spicy sauce, 200-01*
    See also clams; mussels; oysters;
        shrimp
seaweed
    hair, dried, 56
    shrimp wrapped in, 199-200
selenium, 43
sesame
    dressing, broccoli with, 159-60
    oil, 40, 45, 57-58, 159
    seeds, 55
Seven Emotions, 19-21
shallots, 55
shan yao (Chinese yam), 112
sha ren (grains of paradise), 117

she chuang dze (Cnidium monnieri), 79
she chuang dze tang (Cnidium Decoction), 79
shellfish. *See* seafood
Sheng Cycle, 16
shrimp
  basil coconut soup with peppermint sprigs, 143-44
  custard, steamed, with garlic chives and, 211-12
  healing properties of, 39
  wrapped in seaweed, 199-200
sinus infection, 132-33
  Chinese medicine, 133
  healing recipes, 133, 165, 187, 209
  Western medicine, 132-33
Six Evils, 17-19
sleep disturbance. *See* insomnia
smoking, 69-70, 76
soba noodles, with mustard greens, 177-78
Solomon's seal, 115
soup
  basil coconut, with peppermint sprigs, 143-44
  beef essence, 145
  chicken, ginseng, 147
  chicken broth, white fungus in, 152-53
  congee, basic (rice gruel), 173-74
  fishball, 146-47
  hot and sour, vegetarian, 148-49
  melon, winter, 153-54
  soba noodles with mustard greens, 177-78
  spinach and bean curd, 149-50
  sweet potato, 150-51
  tomato and ginger, cold, 151-52
sour foods, 34
soybeans
  chili paste, Szechuan, 51-52
  healing properties of, 43
  sprouts with beef, 182-83
soy sauce, 58
spearmint
  fishball soup, 146-47
  healing properties of, 97, 146

spices
  in Chinese cooking, 53-55
  See also five-spice
spinach
  healing properties of, 149
  soup, and bean curd, 149-50
spleen-pancreas deficiency
  in anemia, 66
  causes of disease, 18, 20, 66
  in diabetes, 90, 91
  in diarrhea, 93
  and diet, 31, 37, 39, 66-67, 91, 99, 108
  and Five Elements system, 15
  in flatulence, 98-99
  in hemorrhoids, 107, 108
  in hepatitis, 110
  in indigestion, 31, 117
  in nausea, 126
sprouts. *See* bean sprouts
squash
  healing properties of, 129, 167
  silk, with oyster sauce, 167
squid with thin wheat noodles in spicy sauce, 200-01
star anise, 55
starwort, yellow, 77
steamers and steaming, 49-50, 58
stir-frying, 58-59
stomach
  causes of disease, 18, 19, 20
  and Five Elements system, 15, 16
  and flatulence, 99
  and nutrition, 31, 37
stomachache, healing recipe for, 193-94
stress, 20, 105, 111, 116, 118, 131
stroke, 18, 88
sulforaphane, 43
sweet foods, 33-34
sweet potato(es)
  healing properties of, 150
  soup, 150-51
swiss chard ribbons, with kohlrabi, 164

T

tan hsiang (sandalwood), 79
Tao (the Way), 10

taro root
  braised with nam yue, 168
  in Chinese cooking, 56-57
  healing properties of, 168
tea
  as breath freshener, 75
  for bronchitis, 77
  chamomile, 92
  cinnamon ginger, 71
  for common cold, 85
  for diarrhea, 92
  ginger, 142
  green, 141-42
  healing properties of, 141
  for herpes, 112
  tannin-containing, 66
thrush, 78
tien ma gou teng yin (Gastrodia and
    Uncaria Beverage), 115
tinctures, herbal, 27
tofu. *See* bean curd
tomato
  healing properties of, 38, 151
  soup, and ginger, cold, 151-52
tongue, in diagnostic process, 21-22
traditional Chinese medicine (TCM).
    See Chinese medicine
tryptophan, 118
turnips, 43

U
ulcers, causes of, 20
unsaturated fats, 45-46
uric acid, 68, 69, 70, 72
urinary tract infection, 134-35
  Chinese medicine, 135
  healing recipes, 135, 150, 153, 179,
    181
  Western medicine, 134-35

V
vaginitis, 78
vegetables
  in Chinese cooking, 55-57
  chlorophyll in, 158
  healing properties of, 37-38, 43,
    158

healing recipes, 155-68
legumes, 36-37
nightshade family, 69
nutrients in, 65
phytochemicals in, 43
See also names of vegetables
vegetarian diet, 65
vitamin A, 69, 96, 121, 131, 133, 149,
    167
vitamin B_{12}, 39, 65
vitamin B/B complex, 44, 69, 79, 81,
    94, 100, 111, 124, 131
vitamin C, 43, 66, 69, 76, 85, 96, 103,
    131, 133, 151, 168
vitamin D, 121, 131
vitamin E, 43, 69, 111, 121, 122, 124,
    131
vitamins
  antioxidants, 43, 85, 100
  fat-soluble, 45
  mail-order sources for, 217
  supplements, 65
vomiting, 18, 75, 91, 95, 104, 108
  and nausea, 125-26

W
walnuts, chicken with, 206-07
water chestnuts, 57, 83, 190-91, 202
Water element, 15, 16, 72
water intake, 35, 41, 87, 134
water retention, 26, 123
Way, the *(Tao),* 10
weight loss, 69, 72, 81
Western medicine
  and anemia, 64-65
  and arthritis, 67-69
  and back pain, 64-66
  and bad breath, 74
  and bronchitis, 75-77
  and candidiasis, 78-79
  vs Chinese medicine, 8-9
  and chronic fatigue syndrome, 80-81
  and common cold, 84-85
  and constipation, 87
  and diabetes, 89-90
  and diarrhea, 92
  and dizziness, 94-95

and ear infections, 96
and flatulence, 97-98
and flu, 100
and hay fever, 102-03
and headache, 104-05
and hemorrhoids, 106-07
and hepatitis, 108-09
and herpes simplex type 2, 111
and hypertension, 113-14
and indigestion, 116-17
and insomnia, 118-19
and menopausal symptoms, 120-21
and menstrual problems, 123-24
and nausea, 125-26
and pain (chronic), 127-29
and psoriasis, 130-31
and sinus infection, 132-33
and urinary tract infection, 134-35
See also nutrition and diet, Western
wind (yang), 18
winter melon. *See* Melon
wok, 50, 58
wolfberry, Chinese, 79
wontons, fish-filled, 190-91
Wood element, 15-16, 20
worrying, cause of disease, 20

Wu Hsing (Five Elements system),
13-16

X
xin yi qingfei yin (Modified Decoction
of Magnolia Flower), 83

Y
yam
braised with nam yue, 168
healing properties of, 38, 168
yeast overgrowth. *See* candidiasis
*Yellow Emperor's Classic of Internal
Medicine, The,* 9, 12, 14, 20
yi mu tsao (leonurus), 124
yin/yang
balance of, 10-12, 34
and diagnostic process, 24-25
disharmony in, 18
of foods, 32-33
yoga, 119, 124
yogurt, 79, 98, 117
yu ju (Solomon's seal), 115

Z
zinc, 43, 66, 69, 85, 100, 131, 133

About the Authors

Rosa Lo San is a cookbook author, chef, and caterer. She has taught courses in Chinese cuisine at cooking schools and to private groups and is a consultant to the food industry. Her articles have appeared in national magazines, including *Food and Wine,* and she has written two cookbooks using her married name, Rosa Lo San Ross: *365 Ways to Cook Chinese* and *Beyond Bok Choy: A Cook's Guide to Asian Vegetables.* As an Asian who grew up in Hong Kong and has lived in America for many years, she has had a longstanding interest in the healing power of Chinese foods.

Suzanne LeVert is a health and medical writer who has authored or coauthored more than a dozen health and medical books. In recent years she has developed a special interest in nutrition as well as holistic or alternative health topics.

Susan Weed
Menopausal yrs

Printed in the United States
47723LVS00006B/64-81